M000013669

FREE Test Taking Tips DVD Offer

Don't forget that doing well on your exam includes both understanding the test content and understanding how to use what you know to do well on the test. We offer a completely FREE Test Taking Tips DVD that covers world class test taking tips that you can use to be even more successful when you are taking your test.

All that we ask is that you email us your feedback about your study guide. To get your **FREE Test Taking Tips DVD**, email freedvd@studyguideteam.com with "FREE DVD" in the subject line and the following information in the body of the email:

- The title of your study guide.
- Your product rating on a scale of 1-5, with 5 being the highest rating.
- Your feedback about the study guide. What did you think of it?
- Your full name and shipping address to send your free DVD.

HESI A2 Study Guide 2019 Pocket Guide

HESI Admission Assessment Exam Review & Practice Test Questions for the HESI 4th Edition Exam

Table of Contents

Quick Overview 1

Test-Taking Strategies 3

Introduction... 12

Math 15

Reading Comprehension 43

Vocabulary.. 56

Grammar 68

Biology... 77

Chemistry 95

Anatomy and Physiology 128

Quick Overview

As you draw closer to taking your exam, effective preparation becomes more and more important. Thankfully, you have this study guide to help you get ready. Use this guide to help keep your studying on track and refer to it often.

This study guide contains several key sections that will help you be successful on your exam. The guide contains tips for what you should do the night before and the day of the test. Also included are test-taking tips. Knowing the right information is not always enough. Many well-prepared test takers struggle with exams. These tips will help equip you to accurately read, assess, and answer test questions.

A large part of the guide is devoted to showing you what content to expect on the exam and to helping you better understand that content. In this guide are practice test questions so that you can see how well you have grasped the content. Then, answer explanations are provided so that you can understand why you missed certain questions.

Don't try to cram the night before you take your exam. This is not a wise strategy for a few reasons. First, your retention of the information will be low. Your time would be better used by reviewing information you already know rather than trying to learn a lot of new information. Second, you will likely become stressed as you try to gain a large amount of knowledge in a short amount of time. Third, you will be depriving yourself of sleep. So be sure to go to bed at a reasonable time the night before. Being well-rested helps you focus and remain calm.

Be sure to eat a substantial breakfast the morning of the exam. If you are taking the exam in the afternoon, be sure to have a good lunch as well. Being hungry is distracting and can make it difficult to focus. You have hopefully spent lots of time preparing for the exam. Don't let an empty stomach get in the way of success!

When travelling to the testing center, leave earlier than needed. That way, you have a buffer in case you experience any delays. This will help you remain calm and will keep you from missing your appointment time at the testing center.

Be sure to pace yourself during the exam. Don't try to rush through the exam. There is no need to risk performing poorly on the exam just so you can leave the testing center early. Allow yourself to use all of the allotted time if needed.

Remain positive while taking the exam even if you feel like you are performing poorly. Thinking about the content you should have mastered will not help you perform better on the exam.

Once the exam is complete, take some time to relax. Even if you feel that you need to take the exam again, you will be well served by some down time before you begin studying again. It's often easier to convince yourself to study if you know that it will come with a reward!

Test-Taking Strategies

1. Predicting the Answer

When you feel confident in your preparation for a multiple-choice test, try predicting the answer before reading the answer choices. This is especially useful on questions that test objective factual knowledge. By predicting the answer before reading the available choices, you eliminate the possibility that you will be distracted or led astray by an incorrect answer choice. You will feel more confident in your selection if you read the question, predict the answer, and then find your prediction among the answer choices. After using this strategy, be sure to still read all of the answer choices carefully and completely. If you feel unprepared, you should not attempt to predict the answers. This would be a waste of time and an opportunity for your mind to wander in the wrong direction.

2. Reading the Whole Question

Too often, test takers scan a multiple-choice question, recognize a few familiar words, and immediately jump to the answer choices. Test authors are aware of this common impatience, and they will sometimes prey upon it. For instance, a test author might subtly turn the question into a negative, or he or she might redirect the focus of the question right at the end. The only way to avoid falling into these traps is to read the entirety of the question carefully before reading the answer choices.

3. Looking for Wrong Answers

Long and complicated multiple-choice questions can be intimidating. One way to simplify a difficult multiple-choice question is to eliminate all of the answer choices that are clearly wrong. In most sets of answers, there will be at least one selection that can be dismissed right away. If the test is administered on paper, the test taker could draw a line through it to indicate that it may be ignored; otherwise, the test taker will have to perform this operation mentally or on scratch paper. In either case, once the obviously incorrect answers have been eliminated, the remaining choices may be considered. Sometimes identifying the clearly wrong answers will give the test taker some information about the correct answer. For instance, if one of the remaining answer choices is a direct opposite of one of the eliminated answer choices, it may well be the correct answer. The opposite of obviously wrong is obviously right! Of course, this is not always the case. Some answers are obviously incorrect simply because they are irrelevant to the question being asked. Still, identifying and eliminating some incorrect answer choices is a good way to simplify a multiple-choice question.

4. Don't Overanalyze

Anxious test takers often overanalyze questions. When you are nervous, your brain will often run wild, causing you to make associations and discover clues that don't actually exist. If you feel that this may be a problem for you, do whatever you can to slow down during the test. Try taking a deep breath or counting to ten. As you read and consider the question, restrict yourself to the particular words used by the author. Avoid thought tangents about what the author *really* meant, or what he or she was *trying* to say. The only things that matter on a multiple-choice test are the words that are actually in the question. You must avoid reading too much into a multiple-choice question, or supposing that the writer meant something other than what he or she wrote.

5. No Need for Panic

It is wise to learn as many strategies as possible before taking a multiple-choice test, but it is likely that you will come across a few questions for which you simply don't know the answer. In this situation, avoid panicking. Because most multiple-choice tests include dozens of questions, the relative value of a single wrong answer is small. As much as possible, you should compartmentalize each question on a multiple-choice test. In other words, you should not allow your feelings about one question to affect your success on the others. When you find a question that you either don't understand or don't know how to answer, just take a deep breath and do your best. Read the entire question slowly and carefully. Try rephrasing the question a couple of different ways. Then, read all of the answer choices carefully. After eliminating obviously wrong answers, make a selection and move on to the next question.

6. Confusing Answer Choices

When working on a difficult multiple-choice question, there may be a tendency to focus on the answer choices that are the easiest to understand. Many people, whether consciously or not, gravitate to the answer choices that require the least concentration, knowledge, and memory. This is a mistake.

When you come across an answer choice that is confusing, you should give it extra attention. A question might be confusing because you do not know the subject matter to which it refers. If this is the case, don't eliminate the answer before you have affirmatively settled on another. When you come across an answer choice of this type, set it aside as you look at the remaining choices. If you can confidently assert that one of the other choices is correct, you can leave the confusing answer aside. Otherwise, you will need to take a moment to try to better understand the confusing answer choice. Rephrasing is one way to tease out the sense of a confusing answer choice.

7. Your First Instinct

Many people struggle with multiple-choice tests because they overthink the questions. If you have studied sufficiently for the test, you should be prepared to trust your first instinct once you have carefully and completely read the question and all of the answer choices. There is a great deal of research suggesting that the mind can come to the correct conclusion very quickly once it has obtained all of the relevant information. At times, it may seem to you as if your intuition is working faster even than your reasoning mind. This may in fact be true. The knowledge you obtain while studying may be retrieved from your subconscious before you have a chance to work out the associations that support it. Verify your instinct by working out the reasons that it should be trusted.

8. Key Words

Many test takers struggle with multiple-choice questions because they have poor reading comprehension skills. Quickly reading and understanding a multiple-choice question requires a mixture of skill and experience. To help with this, try jotting down a few key words and phrases on a piece of scrap paper. Doing this concentrates the process of reading and forces the mind to weigh the relative importance of the question's parts. In selecting words and phrases to write down, the test taker thinks about the question more deeply and carefully. This is especially true for multiple-choice questions that are preceded by a long prompt.

9. Subtle Negatives

One of the oldest tricks in the multiple-choice test writer's book is to subtly reverse the meaning of a question with a word like *not* or *except*. If you are not paying attention to each word in the question, you can easily be led astray by this trick. For instance, a common question format is, "Which of the following is…?" Obviously, if the question instead is, "Which of the following is not…?," then the answer will be quite different. Even worse, the test makers are aware of the potential for this mistake and will include one answer choice that would be correct if the question were not negated or reversed. A test taker who misses the reversal will find what he or she believes to be a correct answer and will be so confident that he or she will fail to reread the question and discover the original error. The only way to avoid this is to practice a wide variety of multiple-choice questions and to pay close attention to each and every word.

10. Reading Every Answer Choice

It may seem obvious, but you should always read every one of the answer choices! Too many test takers fall into the habit of scanning the question and assuming that they understand the question because they recognize a few key words. From there, they pick the first answer choice that answers the question they believe they have read. Test takers who read all of the answer choices might discover that one of the latter answer choices is actually *more* correct. Moreover, reading all of the answer choices can remind you of facts related to the question that can help you arrive at the correct answer. Sometimes, a misstatement or incorrect detail in one of the latter answer choices will trigger your memory of the subject and will enable you to find the right answer. Failing to read all of the answer choices is like not reading all of the items on a restaurant menu: you might miss out on the perfect choice.

11. Spot the Hedges

One of the keys to success on multiple-choice tests is paying close attention to every word. This is never truer than with words like almost, most, some, and sometimes. These words are called "hedges" because they indicate that a statement is not totally true or not true in every place and time. An absolute statement will contain no hedges, but in many subjects, the answers are not always straightforward or absolute. There are always exceptions to the rules in these subjects. For this reason, you should favor those multiple-choice questions that contain hedging language. The presence of qualifying words indicates that the author is taking special care with his or her words, which is certainly important when composing the right answer. After all, there are many ways to be wrong, but there is only one way to be right! For this reason, it is wise to avoid answers that are absolute when taking a multiple-choice test.

An absolute answer is one that says things are either all one way or all another. They often include words like *every*, *always*, *best*, and *never*. If you are taking a multiple-choice test in a subject that doesn't lend itself to absolute answers, be on your guard if you see any of these words.

12. Long Answers

In many subject areas, the answers are not simple. As already mentioned, the right answer often requires hedges. Another common feature of the answers to a complex or subjective question are qualifying clauses, which are groups of words that subtly modify the meaning of the sentence. If the question or answer choice describes a rule to which there are exceptions or the subject matter is complicated, ambiguous, or confusing, the correct answer will require many words in order to be expressed clearly and accurately. In essence, you should not be deterred by answer choices that seem excessively long. Oftentimes, the author of the text will not be able to write the correct answer without offering some qualifications and modifications. Your job is to read the answer choices thoroughly and completely and to select the one that most accurately and precisely answers the question.

13. Restating to Understand

Sometimes, a question on a multiple-choice test is difficult not because of what it asks but because of how it is written. If this is the case, restate the question or answer choice in different words. This process serves a couple of important purposes. First, it forces you to concentrate on the core of the question. In order to rephrase the question accurately, you have to understand it well. Rephrasing the question will concentrate your mind on the key words and ideas. Second, it will present the information to your mind in a fresh way. This process may trigger your memory and render some useful scrap of information picked up while studying.

14. True Statements

Sometimes an answer choice will be true in itself, but it does not answer the question. This is one of the main reasons why it is essential to read the question carefully and completely before proceeding to the answer choices. Too often, test takers skip ahead to the answer choices and look for true statements. Having found one of these, they are content to select it without reference to the question above. Obviously, this provides an easy way for test makers to play tricks. The savvy test taker will always read the entire question before turning to the answer choices. Then, having settled on a correct answer choice, he or she will refer to the original question and ensure that the selected answer is relevant. The mistake of choosing a correct-but-irrelevant answer choice is especially common on questions related to specific pieces of objective knowledge. A prepared test taker will have a wealth of factual knowledge at his or her disposal, and should not be careless in its application.

15. No Patterns

One of the more dangerous ideas that circulates about multiple-choice tests is that the correct answers tend to fall into patterns. These erroneous ideas range from a belief that B and C are the most common right answers, to the idea that an unprepared test-taker should answer "A-B-A-C-A-D-A-B-A." It cannot be emphasized enough that pattern-seeking of this type is exactly the WRONG way to approach a multiple-choice test. To begin with, it is highly unlikely that the test maker will plot the correct answers according to some predetermined pattern. The questions are scrambled and delivered in a random order. Furthermore, even if the test maker was following a pattern in the assignation of correct answers, there is no reason why the test taker would know which pattern he or she was using. Any attempt to discern a pattern in the answer choices is a waste of time and a distraction from the real work of taking the test. A test taker would be much better served by extra preparation before the test than by reliance on a pattern in the answers.

Introduction

Function of the Test

The Health Education Systems, Inc. (HESI) Admission Assessment (A2) Exam is an entrance exam intended for high school graduates seeking admission to post-secondary health programs such as nursing schools. Test-takers have typically not received any training in specific medical subjects. The test is offered nationwide by the colleges and universities that require it as part of an applicant's admission package.

Test Administration

Many of the specifics of the process of HESI administration are determined at the discretion of the testing institution. For instance, each school may choose to administer the entire HESI exam or any portion thereof. Accordingly, there is no set process or schedule for taking the exam; instead, the schedule is determined on a case-by-case basis by the institution administering the exam. Likewise, the cost of the HESI is set by the administering institution. The typical cost is usually around $40-$70.

Find out ahead of time which sections you will be required to take so that you can focus your studying on those areas.

Retesting is generally permitted by HESI, but individual schools may have their own rules on the subject. Likewise, individual schools may set their own policies on whether section scores from different sessions of the HESI can be combined to get one score, or whether a score must come from one coherent session. Students with disabilities may seek accommodations from the schools administering the exam.

Test Format

The exam can include up to eight academic sections with the following distribution of questions:

Section	# of Questions
Mathematics	50
Reading Comprehension	50
Vocabulary	50
Grammar	50
Biology	25
Chemistry	25
Anatomy & Physiology	25
Physics	25

Additionally, there is a Personality Profile and Learning Style Assessment that may be included. Like the academic sections, schools can pick and choose whether to include one, both, or neither of these assessments. Each takes about 15 minutes, and you do not need to study for them.

Scoring

Prospective students and their educational institutions both receive detailed score reports after a prospective applicant completes the exam. Individual student reports include scoring explanations and breakdowns by topic for incorrect answers. The test taker's results can also include study tips based on the individual's Learning Style assessment and identification of the test taker's dominant personality type, strengths, weaknesses, and suggested learning techniques, based on the Personality Profile.

There is no set passing score for the HESI. Instead, individual schools set their own requirements and processes for incorporating scores into admissions decisions. However, HESI recommends that RN and HP programs require a 75% score to pass, and that LPN/LVN programs require a 70% score to pass.

Math

Basic Addition and Subtraction

In order to manipulate numbers through addition and subtraction (also called finding a sum or a difference), an understanding of the value of each number is important.

Addition uses grouping singular units to carry over into the next size of units, while **subtraction** uses removing these units by borrowing from the unit of the next size. Each of these units is a placeholder so the number of units can be tracked or recorded. Traditional addition and subtraction is base ten (10), so once ten units have been collected, this needs to be tallied, in order to start another count to ten.

There are set columns for addition and subtraction: ones, tens, hundreds, thousands, ten-thousands, hundred-thousands, millions, and so on. In order to add or subtract how many units there are total, each column needs to be referenced with the column next to it, starting from the right, or the ONES column.

Every 10 units in the ONES column equals 1 in the TENS column, and every 10 units in the TENS column equals 1 in the HUNDREDS column, and so on. To add or subtract numbers, the units place of each number needs to be lined up. Adding or subtracting starts with the column furthest to the right and then progresses to the left.

What is the sum of 1112, 301, and 527?

    a. 930

    b. 940

    c. 1930

    d. 1940

Explanation

Choice *D* shows the correct addition of the numbers as is required in the following set up:

$$
\begin{array}{r}
1112 \\
527 \\
+301 \\
\hline
1940
\end{array}
$$

The farthest numbers on the right (ONES column) total ten; therefore there is a carry-over to the TENS column, which is the next column to the left. Choice *A* and Choice *C* do not carry-over the one to the TENS column making the column incorrect. Choice *A* and Choice *B* also neglect to carry down the value in the THOUSANDS place, which is a "1."

Basic Multiplication

Multiplication is a method of keeping track of how many times sets of numbers are combined. If the number 6 were to be combined 3 times, it would result in an answer—called the **product**—of 18. The same is true for the number 3 combined 6 times. The order of elements has no bearing on the outcome in multiplication, therefore 3×6 would have the same result as 6×3.

$3 + 3 + 3 + 3 + 3 + 3 = 18$ combining 3, 6 times

OR

$6 + 6 + 6 = 18$ combining 6, 3 times

Properly lining up the numbers on the right can ease the process when multiplying larger numbers. The number with the most digits should be positioned on top and the number with the least digits is placed on the bottom. If both numbers have the same number of digits, select either one for the top or for the bottom. Line up the numbers and begin by multiplying the numbers in the far-right column. If the answer to a column is more than 9, the ones digit will be written below that column and the tens digit will carry to the top of the next column to be added to that column of digits after multiplication. Write the answer below that column, then move to the next column to the left on the top, and multiply it by the same far right column on the bottom. Keep moving to the left one column at a time on the top number until you reach the end. If there is more than one column to the bottom number, you will need to move to the row below the first strand of answers, mark a "0" in the far-right column, and then begin the multiplication process again with the far-right column on top and the second column from the right on the bottom. For each digit in the bottom number there will be a row of answers, each padded with the respective number of zeros on the right. Finally, add up all of the answer rows for one total solution.

What is 425×13?

    a. 5525

    b. 5515

    c. 1700

    d. 1690

Explanation

Choice *A* is the correct solution gained by utilizing the following set up:

Line up the numbers (more digits on top) to multiply.

$$
\begin{array}{r}
\mathbf{425} \\
\mathbf{\times 13} \\
\hline
\end{array}
$$

Begin with the right column on top and the right column on bottom (5×3).

$$
\begin{array}{r}
\mathbf{42}^1 5 \\
\mathbf{\times 1} \ 3 \\
\hline
5
\end{array}
$$

Move one column left on top and multiply by the far-right column on the bottom (2×3).

Remember to add the carry over after you multiply:
$(2 \times 3 = 6, 6 + 1 = 7)$

```
  4 2 ¹5
  × 1  3
  ─────
    7 5
```

Move one column left on top and multiply by the far-right column on the bottom (4×3).
Since this is the last digit on top, write the whole answer below.

```
  4 2 5
  × 1 3
  ─────
1 2 7 5
```

Starting on the far-right column, on top, repeat this pattern for the next number left on the bottom.

```
  4 2 5
  × 1 3
  ─────
1 2 7 5
    5 0
```

Write the answers below the first line of answers, remember to begin with a zero place-holder. Continue the pattern.

```
  4 2 5
  × 1 3
  ─────
1 2 7 5
  2 5 0
```

Since this is the last digit on top, write the whole answer below.

$$\begin{array}{r} 4\,2\,5 \\ \times\,1\,3 \\ \hline 1\,2\,7\,5 \\ 4\,2\,5\,0 \end{array}$$

Now add the answer rows together; pay attention to make sure they are still correctly aligned.

$$\begin{array}{r} 4\,2\,5 \\ \times\,1\,3 \\ \hline 1\,2\,7\,5 \\ 4\,2\,5\,0 \\ \hline 5\,5\,2\,5 \end{array}$$

Choice *B* does not carry the digit when multiplying into the tens position. Choice *C* does not utilize a zero for a place-holder when tabulating the second row of numbers. Choice *D* makes the mistake in not carrying the digit in the multiplication and not using a zero place-holder for the second row of multiplication.

Basic Division

Division uses the repeating process of an algorithm to solve a problem. **Division** expresses how many times a number (divisor) can evenly go into another number (**dividend**). This process can be done through lining up the two numbers and organizing the results to get an answer (**quotient**).

Lining up the divisor to be divided into the dividend assists in matching smaller portions of both numbers for division and giving a systematic approach to solving the entire problem.

Set up the problem with the divisor being divided into the dividend and check for divisibility into the first digit of the numerator. If it is divisible by a whole number, mark that number over top; otherwise, include the next number to the right in the dividend. Repeat this process until there is a whole number above the appropriate place in the dividend. Then multiply the two numbers used so far, with the answer written under the dividend. Subtract the portion of the dividend used by the product of the multiplication. Drop down the next number place from the original dividend to the ones place of the difference and begin the entire process again.

Question

What is 1,092 divided by 42?

    a. 24
    b. 26
    c. 32
    d. 36

Explanation

Choice *B* is the correct answer, as detailed below. Choice *A*, Choice *C*, and Choice *D* all involve a miscalculation during the division process.

Check for divisibility into the first unit of the numerator, 1.

$$42 \overline{) 1092}$$

42 cannot go into 1, so add on the next unit in the denominator, 0.

$$42\overline{)1092}$$

42 cannot go into 10, so add on the next unit in the denominator, 9.

$$42\overline{)1092}$$

42 can be divided into 109, 2 times. Write the 2 over the 9 in 109 and multiply 42×2, which is 84.

Write the 84 under 109 for subtraction and note the remainder, 25, is less than 42.

$$42\overline{)1092} \\ 84 \\ 25$$

Drop down the next digit in the numerator to create a number 42 can divide intonow repeat the steps above.

42 divides into 252 six times write the 6 over the 0 and multiply 42×6, which is 252.

$$
\begin{array}{r}
2 \\
42\overline{\smash{)}1092} \\
84 \\
\hline
252 \\
\end{array}
$$

Write the 252 under 252 for subtraction and note there is no remainder.

$$
\begin{array}{r}
26 \\
42\overline{\smash{)}1092} \\
84 \\
\hline
252 \\
252 \\
\end{array}
$$

Thus, the solution is 26.

Decimals

Decimals mark the division between the whole portion and the fractional (or decimal) portion of a number. A number such as 345 is a whole number, but there is still a decimal place. The decimal place in 345 is to the right of the 5, but usually not written, since there is no fractional or decimal portion to this number. The same number can be written as 345.0 or 345.00 or 345.000, etc. Zeros to the right of the decimal place can be

23

dropped so long as there are no other digits after them. For example, 27.0500000 can be written as 27.05 but not 27 because the 5 two places to the right of the decimal point represents five hundredths and is part of the value of the number.

The position of the decimal place can change the entire value of a number and impact calculations. When asked to round to a certain decimal place, it is important to know which one is being referenced. In the United States, the decimal place is also used when representing money. Since each decimal place is a factor of ten, an accident in proper decimal point placement could result in significant errors like accidentally giving someone $200.00 instead of $20.00!

The next page is a review of decimal place names.

Table of the decimal place names with a decimal and arrow in the middle between ones and tenths

Ten-thousands	Thousands	Hundreds	Tens	Ones	Tenths	Hundredths	Thousandths	Ten-thousandths

Decimal

What number is in the hundredths place in 12,436.897?

    a. 2

    b. 4

    c. 9

    d. 7

Explanation

Choice *C* is the correct answer. Referring to the chart provided above, the hundredths place matches up with the second number to the right of the decimal place, which is 9 in 12,436.897. Choice *A* is in the thousands place (third position to the left of the decimal), Choice *B* is in the hundreds place (second position to the left of the decimal), and Choice *D* is in the thousandths place (third position to the right of the decimal).

Fractions

Fractions represent whole numbers that have been divided into a certain number of equal-sized parts. The numerator, which is the number above the fraction bar, represents the part, while the denominator, which is the number on bottom, represents the whole amount. For example, the fraction $\frac{1}{4}$ represents one quarter of a whole. Essentially, it can be visualized as a pizza cut into four equal quarters and then one piece is taken. That piece is $\frac{1}{4}$ of the pizza. If the same pizza was cut into 8 slices and two were taken, $\frac{2}{8}$ of the pizza would be gone. These two slices together are actually the same amount as $\frac{1}{4}$, just not in reduced, or simplified, form. The greatest common factor of both the numerator and denominator should always be divided out so that a fraction is reduced.

When the numerator of a fraction is less than the denominator, such as $\frac{3}{5}$, the fraction is considered a proper fraction. When the numerator is greater than the denominator, such as $\frac{8}{3}$, the fraction is considered an improper fraction. When there is a whole number combined with a proper fraction, such as $2\frac{1}{3}$, it is considered to be a mixed number. A mixed number can be converted to an improper fraction by multiplying the integer by the denominator, adding that calculated product to the numerator, and dividing the calculated sum by the original denominator. For example:

$$2\frac{1}{3} = \frac{2 \times 3 + 1}{3} = \frac{7}{3}$$

Because dividing by zero is undefined, the denominator of a fraction can never be zero.

Question
What is the numerator when $\frac{28}{42}$ is reduced?

    a. 2
    b. 3
    c. 4
    d. 7

Explanation
Choice A is correct as 2 would be the numerator when the fraction is reduced. The greatest common factor of 28 and 42 is 14. 14 goes into 28 twice and into 42 three times. Therefore, $\frac{28}{42}$

reduced is $\frac{2}{3}$, which means that the numerator (the top number) is 2.

Multiplication of Fractions

The multiplication of fractions is simpler if they are lined up correctly. Once set next to each other, multiply the numerators across the top, resulting in the upper value of the fraction, then multiply the denominators across the bottom, resulting in the lower value of the fraction. The new fraction might need to be reduced. A fraction can be reduced if the same number can evenly be divided into both the numerator and the denominator. Reducing fractions can also be performed before the multiplication is executed through cross-reduction, which reduces the work needed at the end.

Question

What is $\frac{4}{5} \times \frac{9}{10}$? Give your answer in reduced form.

 a. $\frac{17}{10}$

 b. $\frac{18}{25}$

 c. $\frac{36}{50}$

 d. $\frac{40}{45}$

<u>Explanation</u>
Choice *B* is given in the proper reduced form, as shown below:

Line up the fractions with numerators on top and denominators on the bottom:

$$\frac{4}{5} \times \frac{9}{10}$$

Multiply across the top and across the bottom:

$$\frac{4 \times 9}{5 \times 10}$$

Reduce the fraction:

$$\frac{36}{50}$$

For this example, 2 evenly divides into both the numerator and denominator.

$$36 \div 2 = 18$$

$$50 \div 2 = 25$$

$$= \frac{18}{25}$$

OR reducing can also be executed during the initial set up, before the multiplication takes place, as shown here:

Line up the reduced fractions, then multiply across the top and across the bottom.

$$\frac{\cancel{4}^{\,2}}{5} \times \frac{9}{\cancel{10}_{\,5}}$$

Choice *A* shows the addition of the two fractions, Choice *C* is not reduced, and Choice *D* involves a miscalculation when cross-multiplying the fractions.

Division of Fractions

Division of fractions is just like the multiplication with two small differences. The first difference is that the order of the fractions matters and should not be changed from the original problem. The other difference is that the second fraction (divisor) is inverted (flip the numerator and denominator, which is called the **reciprocal**) before multiplying or reducing can be performed.

The following is an example:

<u>Question</u>
What is $\frac{12}{15} \div \frac{2}{3}$? Give your answer in reduced form.

    a. $\frac{6}{5}$

    b. $\frac{4}{7}$

    c. $\frac{24}{45}$

    d. $\frac{36}{30}$

Explanation

Choice *A* is correct, as detailed below:

Line up the fractions:

$$\frac{12}{15} \div \frac{2}{3}$$

Invert the second fraction and change to multiplication:

$$\frac{12}{15} \times \frac{3}{2}$$

Multiply across the top and across the bottom:

$$\frac{12 \times 3}{15 \times 2}$$

Reduce by dividing both numbers by 6:

$$\frac{36}{30}$$

$$= \frac{6}{5}$$

Choice *B* and Choice *C* are miscalculations due to not inverting the fraction and not multiplying the correct numbers. Choice *D* is not reduced.

Changing Fractions to Decimals

To change a fraction into a decimal, divide the numerator by the denominator until there are no remainders. This could involve inserting additional zeros after the decimal place in the dividend. The conversion of a fraction into a decimal can occasionally result in something called a **repeating decimal**, so rounding is often acceptable. A straight line above the repeating portion also denotes that a decimal repeats.

<u>Question</u>
What is $\frac{2}{5}$ written as a decimal?
    a. 0.4
    b. 4.0
    c. 4.4
    d. 40

<u>Explanation</u>
Choice *A* is the correct calculation as shown below:

Set up the division problem.

$$5 \overline{\smash{\big)}\ 2}$$

5 does not go into 2, so place the decimal and insert a zero after it.

$$5 \overline{\smash{\big)}\ 2.0}$$

5 goes into 20 four times, so write a 4 over the zero. There is no remainder, but remember to bring up the decimal point from the dividend to the quotient. The solution is 0.4.

$$
\begin{array}{r}
0.4 \\
5\overline{)2.0} \\
2\,0 \\
\hline
0
\end{array}
$$

Choice *B*, Choice *C*, and Choice *D*, involve miscalculations or incorrect placements of the decimal.

Changing Decimals to Fractions

To change a decimal to a fraction, place the decimal portion of the number, the numerator, over the denominator of the respective place value of the fraction, then reduce, if possible.

For example, to change 0.42 to a fraction, place 42 over 100 (because 0.42 is "forty-two hundredths") and reduce.

$$
\frac{42}{100} = \frac{21}{50}
$$

What is 0.28 written as a reduced fraction?

   a. $\frac{1}{28}$

   b. $\frac{28}{100}$

   c. $\frac{14}{50}$

   d. $\frac{28}{10}$

Explanation

Choice C is the correct conversion. The decimal 0.28 is read as "twenty-eight hundredths," which means $\frac{28}{100}$. This can be reduced by dividing both the numerator and denominator by 2. The result is $\frac{14}{50}$.

Ratios and Proportions

Fractions are closely related to ratios and proportions. Ratios can be adjusted to larger or smaller scales, which is useful for measuring in recipes, chemistry, medicine, etc. Ratios can be adjusted by keeping the same overall proportion of the items being aligned. Any adjustment to one part of a ratio must be done to the other parts to maintain proportionality. Ratios have a minimum of two items being mapped and can have any number as a maximum number of items being connected. The most important thing to remember is if any part of a ratio is altered, then the exact same alteration needs to be applied to all other parts of the ratio.

Question

If a doctor prescribes a 4 to 3 ratio (written 4:3) of saline to water for a patient and there are 8 ounces of saline available, how much water would need to be mixed with the saline to provide the correct proportion to the patient?

  a. 3 ounces
  b. 4 ounces
  c. 6 ounces
  d. 8 ounces

Explanation

Choice *C* is the correct solution for calculating the ratio as shown below:

The original proportion of 4 to 3 means for every 4 parts saline, there need to 3 parts water. It is more simply expressed with numbers, as follows:

Saline : water mixture = 4:3

If there are 8 ounces of saline, there will need to be 6 ounces of water, which is calculated as followed:

In order to get 8 ounces, the 4 was multiplied by 2:

$$4 \times 2 = 8$$

Since the saline has been multiplied by 2, so should the water:

$$3 \times 2 = 6$$

The new ratio would be 8:6; 8 ounces of saline for 6 ounces of water. Choice *A* does not proportionately show any increase to the original value of the second number. Choice *B* and Choice *D* are incorrect calculations of the new proportion.

Percentages

The percentage of a number is another way of finding a proportion of that number. Percentages are out of 100 units. So, 100 percent of something is the entire, whole, unit. To calculate using percentages, a percent is written in proportion to 100. Any given percent is divided by 100 (done by moving the decimal two places to the left) to convert it to a regular number.

To convert a number to a percent, reverse the above and multiply the decimal by 100 (move the decimal two places to the right).

For calculating percentages, the original problem needs to be translated into a math equation to find the solution. Key terms given in the original problem are important. The word "of" means to multiply, "what" or "what number" are the unknown (N), and "is" means equals. These terms can be formed into an equation such as:

Problem:

$$first\ value\ is\ what\ percent\ of\ second\ value$$

Translated into an equation:

$$first\ value = N \times second\ value$$

The following is an example:

Question
8.4 is 20% of what number?

    a. 0.42
    b. 1.68
    c. 42
    d. 168

Explanation
Choice C shows the correct calculation of the value as shown below:

Translate the givens into a math equation:

"Is" means = (equals)

Convert the percent into a useable number:

$$20\% = 0.20$$

"Of "means multiply ($\times$)

"What number" means the unknown (N)

Write out the equation based on the givens:

$$8.4 = 0.20 \ (X)8.4 = 0.20 \times N$$

Divide both sides by 0.20 to get X by itself:

$$\frac{8.4}{0.20} = \frac{0.20 \ N}{0.20}$$

Solve:

$$42 = N$$

Choice *A* misaligns the decimal place, Choice *B* does not divide the numbers correctly and misaligns the decimal place, and Choice *D* does not divide the numbers correctly.

12-hour Clock versus Military Time

When telling time with a regular or 12-hour clock, counting starts at 12 AM-midnight, increasing each hour by whole numbers. 1 AM would be next, 2 AM, 3 AM, and so on. Once the count reaches 12 again (at noon), it becomes 12 PM, and the count goes from 1 PM, 2 PM, 3 PM, and so on. Military time also begins at midnight and continues on to 1, 2, 3 and so on, except it does not use AM or PM because it uses a 24-hour clock. Midnight is actually the 24th hour in the count for military time. The colon is usually not used; so, for example, 6:00 PM on a 12-hour clock is written as 1800, and pronounced "eighteen-hundred hours" in Military time. A small trick to converting from military to regular time is if the original time is 12 hundred hours or less, it is equivalent to AM in regular time. If the original time is 1300 hours or more, subtract 12 and add PM to convert it to regular time.

The following is an example:

Question
A patient requires a dose of medicine at 2300. What time is the equivalent to this on the AM/PM readings?

    a. 3 AM
    b. 3 PM
    c. 11 AM
    d. 11 PM

Explanation
Choice *D* shows the correct conversion as follows:

The original military time is 13 or more, so subtract 12 from the time.

$$23 - 12 = 11 \ (PM)$$

Choice *A* and Choice *B* do not convert the correct number and Choice *C* does not convert to the correct time (AM rather than PM).

Algebra

The term **algebra** describes mathematics that have differing or changeable variables. This term is regularly applied to real-world situations, due to its versatility. Algebra often uses **variables**, which can be of unknown value, or different values for different situations. Variables are usually represented by a letter, such as X or Y. These are helpful placeholders when attempting to solve story problems.

Other basic tips for navigating algebra include the use of shorthand, so that multiplication signs (x) and unknown variables (X) are not confused. Parentheses around an object in an equation signify multiplication. For example, (8)(4) = 8 times 4.

Another shorthand is by eliminating the multiplication sign between numbers and variables; it is understood that they are still multiplied together. So instead of writing 5 multiplied by X as $5 \times X$, it would be written as $5X$.

Question
What is the value of x in $4x + 5 = 25$?
    a. 4
    b. 5
    c. 20
    d. 25

Explanation
Choice *B* is the proper algebraic solution as shown below:

First isolate the term containing x on the left side by subtracting 5 from both sides:

$$4x + 5 - 5 = 25 - 5$$

Next, get the x alone by dividing both sides by 4:

$$\frac{4x}{4} = \frac{20}{4}$$

Solve:

$$x = 5$$

Choice *A*, Choice *C*, and Choice *D* are all miscalculations of the answer.

Helpful Information to Memorize

- 2 Tbsp = 1/8 cup
- 1 fl oz = 30 mL
- 128 fl oz = 8 pt = 16 cup
- 1 gal = 4 qt = 3.79 L
- 1 tsp = 5 mL
- 1 Tbsp = 15 mL
- 1 cup = 250 mL
- 1 qt = 4 cup = 0.95 L
- 28.1 g = 1 oz = 125 mL
- 450 g = 16 oz = 1 lb
- 16 oz = 1 lb
- 12 in = 1 ft
- 3 ft = 1 yd
- 1 mile = 5,280 ft
- 1 mile = 1.61 km

Order of Operations:

1. Parentheses: calculate anything inside parentheses first

2. Exponents: apply any exponents second

3. Multiplication: execute any multiplication

4. Division: execute any division

5. Addition: execute any addition

6. Subtraction: execute any subtraction

The first letters of these operations, in order, form the word
PEMDAS.

<u>Question</u>
What would be the final result of $(3 + 2)(8 \div 2) + 8$

    a. 4
    b. 14
    c. 21
    d. 28

<u>Explanation</u>
Choice *D* shows the proper execution of the order of
operations as shown below:

Calculate the operations inside parentheses first:

$$(3 + 2)(8 \div 2) + 8$$

Then, multiply:

$$(5)(4) + 8$$

Finally, add:

$$20 + 8$$

$$28$$

Choice *A* and Choice *B* make mistakes in calculations,
specifically adding and multiplying before executing the
operations inside the parentheses. Choice *C* multiplies before
executing the operations inside of the parentheses.

Reading Comprehension

Identifying the Main Idea

The **main idea** of a passage is a brief summary of what the passage is about. As an answer choice, the main idea of a passage will probably be around a sentence long and includes the **topic**, or what the passage is about, and the author's argument surrounding the topic. Be sure not to confuse supporting details with the main idea. **Supporting details** are evidence, testimonies, or factual statements that support the main idea. Let's take a look at a main idea question below:

Question

> More than 21 million US adults 18–64 years of age have a disability. These are adults with serious difficulty walking or climbing stairs; hearing; seeing; or concentrating, remembering, or making decisions. Most adults with disabilities are able to participate in physical activity, yet nearly half of them get no aerobic physical activity. Physical activity benefits all adults, whether or not they have a disability, by reducing their risk of serious chronic diseases, such as heart disease, stroke, diabetes, and some cancers. Only 44% of adults with disabilities who visited a doctor in the past year were told by a doctor to get physical activity, yet adults with disabilities were 82% more likely to be physically active if their doctor recommended it.

> "Adults with Disabilities,"
> https://www.cdc.gov/vitalsigns/disabilities/

What is the main purpose of this article?

    a. To persuade the audience to encourage people with disabilities to get physical exercise because their doctors fail to inform them of the health risks that come from a lack of exercise.

    b. To inform the audience of the statistics of how many adults with disabilities engage in physical activities and how many of their doctors recommend it.

    c. To contradict a widespread rumor that people with disabilities get sufficient exercise and are therefore not susceptible to chronic illnesses.

    d. To critique the healthcare system and bring awareness to the fact that doctors never approach illness with a holistic treatment in mind, which would be best for persons with disabilities.

Explanation

Choice *B* is the best answer choice above because it matches the topic (adults with disabilities and their physical activities) with the author's intention (to inform the audience of the facts of the topic). Choice *A* is incorrect because there is not much persuasion going on here. Persuasion usually includes inciting the audience to act in some fashion, and we are not told we should act in any way. Choice *C* is incorrect; the passage says that "nearly half" of adults with disabilities "get no aerobic physical activity," thus debunking the assertion in the answer choice that they are "therefore not susceptible to chronic illnesses." This is opposite of what the passage says. Choice *D* is incorrect; the last few sentences may be a transition to lead into a critique of the healthcare system, but the passage does not offer outright criticism of the healthcare system as a whole.

Identifying Supporting Details

Supporting details are the evidence that offer support for the main idea of a passage. Supporting details may be facts, statistics, examples, testimonies, or any other kind of data that confirms to the audience that the author knows what they are talking about and can prove the argument they have presented. When looking for supporting details in a passage, determine what the author does to prove his or her main argument. Let's look at an example question:

Question

> Contaminated food sent to several states can make people sick with the same germ. These multistate outbreaks cause serious illness, and more of these outbreaks are being found. Multistate outbreaks caused 56% of deaths in all reported foodborne outbreaks, although they accounted for just 3% of all such outbreaks from 2010 to 2014. Foods that cause multistate outbreaks are contaminated before they reach a restaurant or home kitchen. Investigating these outbreaks often reveals problems on the farm, in processing or in distribution that resulted in contaminated food. Lessons learned from these outbreaks are helping make food safer. To protect the public's health, government at all levels and food industries need to work together to stop outbreaks and keep them from happening in the first place.

"Safer Food Saves Lives" Overview,
https://www.cdc.gov/vitalsigns/foodsafety-2015/index.html

Which of the following statements is NOT a detail from the passage?

a. Multistate food outbreaks cause 56% of deaths in all reported foodborne outbreaks.

b. Most foods that cause outbreaks are contaminated before they reach the restaurant or kitchen.

c. There are often problems on the farm, in processing, or in distribution that result in contaminated food.

d. Multistate outbreaks from contaminated food have decreased in the years 2010 to 2014.

Explanation

First let's look for the main idea of the passage. The main idea of the passage is to encourage the government to protect food distribution at all levels to prevent contaminated food-related deaths. To prove that there's an issue with food-related deaths, we have the information from Choice A: Multistate food outbreaks caused 56% of deaths in all reported foodborne outbreaks. Another detail from the passage is Choice B, an explanation of *where* the food is contaminated (before it reaches a restaurant or home kitchen). Finally, the detail in Choice C is also in the passage: there are often problems on the farm, in processing, or in distribution that results in contaminated food. Choice D is a detail that is *not* found in the passage. For supporting details, it's mostly about paying attention to which details are explicitly stated in the passage to support the main idea of the author.

Finding the Meaning of Words in Context

When readers do not know the meaning of a certain word within a passage, taking into consideration the surrounding context is one of the best ways to determine the word's definition. **Context clues**, or hints at the word's meaning in the sentence, can be help elucidate the definition of the unknown word. Context clues may provide a **synonym** (same-meaning word), an **antonym** (opposite-meaning word), a restatement of the word, an example, an explanation, or information pertaining to the word's structure (the word's affixes or etymology). Let's look at an example:

Question

It was the middle of the work week, and Meredith walked into the meeting with a new confidence she had been cultivating over the weekend. She knew that she wanted to inspire her team because they had recently been experiencing setback after setback. They were defeated, and this defeat showed on their faces and in their attitudes surrounding work. After she gave her speech, Meredith hoped that they would **emulate** her confidence rather than disregard the positive opportunities she inspired in the meeting.

What is the meaning of the word "emulate" in the paragraph?
a. Neglect
b. Eschew
c. Imitate
d. Nullify

Explanation

The best choice is *C*, imitate. Meredith hoped they would "imitate" her confidence. If we look at the surrounding context, we can see that we are given an antonym, "disregard," from the key words "rather than," which suggests an opposite reaction to "emulate." Emulate would then mean to pay attention to or mirror something someone else is doing, rather than disregard what they are doing. Choice A, neglect, is the opposite meaning of the word "imitate." Choice B, eschew, means to avoid or ignore. Meredith would not want the team to avoid her confidence after her speech, so this is incorrect. Choice D, nullify, means to cancel or revoke. Cancelling confidence is something Meredith would not want to happen either. The best choice here from the surrounding context is "imitate."

Identifying a Writer's Purpose and Tone

For a reader to determine the author's **purpose** in writing a text, the reader must ask *why* the author wrote what they did. Also, how is the author interacting with his or her audience? Authors can write to entertain, inform, or persuade the audience. Usually if the author is trying to persuade the audience, the author goes beyond informing to try and convince the audience to act in a certain way. If a writer's purpose is to persuade, check to see what his or her angle is and if the writer is being objective or biased (leaning one way without proper objectivity).

A writer's **tone** can be a wide variety of emotions used to affect the audience, such as humor, joy, seriousness, pessimism, optimism, sadness, irony, outrage, anger, or cheerfulness, among others. To determine a writer's tone, pay close attention to the **connotation**, or the feeling that comes from a word used. For example, if a writer is using adjectives like "overbearing" or "cumbersome" to describe someone, he or she is giving off a negative connotation. Likewise, using words like "agreeable" or "pleasant" indicates a positive connotation. Connotation is also a good way to determine if the writer is biased or not towards the subject. Let's look at an example of a tone question:

Question

> New 2010 estimates show that the number of Americans without health insurance is growing, affecting middle-income Americans as well as those living in poverty. About 50 million adults 18–64 years old had no health insurance for at least some of the past 12 months. People in all income brackets have been affected, not just adults living in poverty, according to a 2009 survey. In the past few years, the number of adults aged 18–64 who went without health insurance for at least part of the past 12 months increased by an average of 1.1 million per year. About half of those additional adults were middle-income. Adults without consistent health insurance are more likely to skip medical care because of cost concerns, which can lead to poorer health, higher long-term health care costs, and early death.

From *CDC Vital Signs*,
https://www.cdc.gov/vitalsigns/pdf/2010-11-vitalsigns.pdf

In terms of its tone and form, the passage is most appropriately described as which of the following?
   a. A contemplative claim
   b. An outraged objection
   c. An aloof outline
   d. A fervent argument

Choice *A*, a contemplative claim, is the best answer choice here. The passage is making a claim that the numbers of Americans without health insurance is increasing, and the tone is more thoughtful than outraged, aloof, or fervent. An *outraged* or *fervent* objection or argument would have a much more impassioned tone than this informative text. There are no words that connote any kind of intensity or fury, so Choices *B* and *D* are incorrect. The passage does not display aloofness either. Likewise, it displays informative facts and appropriate concern, so Choice *C* is also incorrect.

Distinguishing Between Fact and Opinion

The difference between fact and opinion is that a **fact** can be proven, and an **opinion** cannot be proven. For example, if I say that Wanda has a silver truck, and I can prove that to be true, then that is a fact. If I say that Wanda's silver truck is ugly, I am sharing my opinion, since the statement does not contain something measurable that can be proven to be true or false. It's important to be able to distinguish between facts and opinion in a passage because doing so will help determine if the author has any underlying assumptions present. **Assumptions** are ideas that the author has about a certain topic that may or may not be grounded in reality.

Let's look at a fact/opinion question below:

As I drove to the hospital with my oldest friend, I knew that this might be the end of her life. She had lymphoma that had spread rapidly in the past six months. Her daughter had just passed away from a drug overdose. She repeatedly said to me the week before that she didn't think she could go on. The drive there seemed like a whole eternity. Although she was in a lot of pain, my friend looked peaceful on the drive there, as if she had courage to face whatever came her way. She was courageous and had changed many people's lives over the course of her own.

Which of the following phrases from the passage is NOT considered a fact?

a. She had lymphoma that had spread rapidly in the past six months.

b. She was courageous and had changed many people's lives over the course of her own.

c. Her daughter had just passed away from a drug overdose.

d. She repeatedly said to me the week before that she didn't think she could go on.

Explanation
Choice *B* is the best answer choice here because it is an opinion, and the rest of the answer choices are based in fact. Choice *A* is a fact; whether or not someone has cancer can be proven to be true or false. Choice *C* is also a fact. Whether or not her daughter passed away can also be proven to be true or

false. Choice *D* is tricky; that the woman *told* the speaker she couldn't go on is a fact; whether or not the woman *could go on* or not was her own opinion. So, we have an opinion within a fact, so to speak, because this was told to the speaker (fact). Choice *B* is an opinion. Others may not think the woman was courageous or that she had changed many people's lives. This is a subjective opinion given by the speaker.

Making Logical Inferences

Inferences are conclusions that can be reached based off of evidence and reasoning. Inferences will never be directly stated in the passage; but they will be ideas that you can assume to be true because of the support that the author gives. An inference is always based on logic and is always a guess, so even if an "inference" isn't mentioned directly in the passage, it doesn't necessarily mean that it isn't there. For example, if I say "I am outside in 100-degree heat in Texas, and all the kids are out of school in the afternoon," one might make the inference that it is summer in Texas. Let's look at what an inference question might look like:

Question

It was the morning before school started, and everything was just about ready for Brianna to walk out of the door. She had her syllabi printed for all the students, her fancy new briefcase, and her lecture notes. Brianna had never done this before, but she was confident in her abilities from the education she had received. Sure, she was nervous; but an overwhelming feeling of excitement filled her up because she knew this was exactly the place she wanted to be. She grabbed her keys, turned off the lights, and headed out the door.

Which of the following can be inferred from the passage?

a. Brianna is taking her daughter to school for the first time.

b. Brianna is a surgeon on her first rotation.

c. Brianna is a student at a prestigious university.

d. Brianna is a lecturer on her way to teach her first class.

Explanation

The best answer is Choice *D*: Brianna is a lecturer on her way to teach her first class. We can infer this to be a logical explanation of the passage because we see that Brianna has "students" and a "syllabi" to show them. She also has a briefcase, not a backpack, implying a professional dress code. Choices *A*, *B*, and *C* are incorrect; the passage does not mention a daughter. There is also no mention of surgery or rotations. And although Brianna is "going to school," she is probably not a student at that school; even if she is, the best answer is Choice *D* because it has the strongest inference that Brianna is going to school to lecture.

Summarizing

A **summary** is a brief statement that embodies the entirety of a text or passage. Summarizing a passage requires a full comprehension of the passage before writing begins. Test takers should read the passage a few times over, if possible, and then write down in one or two sentences the most important points of the passage. Let's look at a summary question:

Question

Dental sealants are thin coatings that when painted on the chewing surfaces of the back teeth (molars) can prevent cavities for many years. School-age children (ages 6-11) without sealants have almost 3 times more 1st molar cavities than those with sealants. Although the overall number of children with sealants has increased over time, low-income children are 20% less likely to have them and 2 times more likely to have untreated cavities than higher-income children. Untreated cavities can cause pain, infection, and problems eating, speaking, and learning. States can help millions more children prevent cavities by starting or expanding programs that offer dental sealants in schools.

"Dental Sealants Prevent Cavities," *CDC*,
https://www.cdc.gov/vitalsigns/dental-sealants/index.html

Which sentence best summarizes the passage?

   a. Children who do not receive dental sealants are 3 times more likely to develop molar cavities than children who do receive dental sealants.

   b. Low income children are more likely to have cavities than high-income children, and this has to change.

   c. Dental sealants help prevent cavities and have the potential of reducing the number of cavities, especially with low-income children.

   d. Those who cannot afford dental sealants are more likely to have cavities, which can cause problems with eating, sleeping, and learning.

Explanation

Choice *C* is the best summary because it includes all the most important details: what sealants are, what they do, and who they can help. Choice *A* is incorrect; the statement is true, but we are only given one specific detail from the passage and not the main points. Choices *B* and *D* also offer specific details from the passage. However, keep in mind that a proper summary will give the main points and leave the details out.

Vocabulary

Root Word

A **root word** is the most basic form of a word, and prefixes and suffixes can be attached to a root word to change the form. For example, the root word *phobia* means fear. When we add a prefix to the word, we can get *arachnophobia* (fear of spiders) or *cynophobia* (fear of dogs). Taking the prefixes away, we are left with the root word *phobia*. Let's look at an example vocabulary question:

Question
What is the best definition of the word <u>dysfunction</u>?
  a. Exacerbate
  b. Abnormality
  c. Dilate
  d. Lethargic

Explanation
For the vocabulary test questions, one way to determine what a vocabulary word means is by looking at the root word and its prefix and/or suffix separately. In the word *dysfunction*, we have the root word *function* and the prefix *dys*. *Function* means to work or operate in a particular way. The prefix *dys* denotes *bad* or *difficult*. Therefore, the word *dysfunction* would mean functioning with difficulty; the word closest to this is *abnormality*, which means the quality or state of being abnormal or defected, which is Choice *B*. Choice *A*, *exacerbate*, means something that becomes more intense in nature. Choice *C*, *dilate*, means to enlarge or extend. Choice *D*, *lethargic*,

means sluggish or apathetic. Let's look at a table of common root words below:

Root	Meaning	Example
bio	life	autobiography
cede, cess	go, yield	procession
celer	fast	deceleration
chron	time	anachronism
claim, clam	shout	exclamatory
cred	believe	incredulous
dict	speak	prediction
form	shape	conformity
funct	work, operate	malfunctioning
graph	writing	autograph
ject	throw	objection
loc	place	dislocated
miss, mit	let go	intermittent
mob, mobi	move	immobile
mut	change	mutation
phon	sound	telephone
pop	people	unpopular
port	carry	transportation
put	think	computation
reg	rule	deregulate
rupt	break	disruption
scrib, script	written	description
sed, sid	sit	residence
spec, spect	see. look	inspection
serv	save, keep	conservation
struct	build	construction
tact, tang	touch	intangible

temp	time	contemporary
ten, tin	hold	detention
vers, vert	turn	introverted
angi	blood vessel	angiogram
audi	hearing	auditory
bio	life	biology
brachi	arm	brachial
carcin	cancer	carcinogen
cardi	heart	cardiology
carp, carpo	wrist	carpal tunnel
cerebr	brain	cerebral
derm	skin	dermatology
dors	back	dorsal
gastro	stomach	gastroenterology
hemato	blood	hematoma
lingu	tongue	sublingual
manu	hand	manuscript
nerv	nerve	nervous system
ocul	eye	ocular
oro	mouth	oropharyngeal
oto	ear	otology
path	disease	pathogen
pulmon	lungs	pulmonary
septo	infection	septic
spir	breathe	respirator
thorac	chest/thorax	thoracentesis
thyro	thyroid gland	thyroid
trach	neck	trachea
umbilic	navel	umbilical cord
ventr	front of body	ventral

Prefix

A **prefix** is an addition at the beginning of a root word. Prefixes attach to root words to tell us more about the root word. For example, the word *abnormal* means *deviating away from the normal*—but why? The prefix *ab* means *away*. Therefore, if we have the word *ab* in front of *normal*, that means it is *away from normal*, or *different from normal*. Let's look at another vocabulary question:

Question
Select the correct meaning of the underlined word in the following sentence.

The nurse measured her <u>sublingual</u> temperature against her axillary temperature.

    a. In the ear
    b. In the rectum
    c. Under the armpit
    d. Under the tongue

Explanation
The correct answer Choice is *D*, under the tongue. The root word of *sublingual* is *lingual,* which means *tongue*. The prefix is *sub*, which means *under*. Therefore, if we pay attention the prefix and how it relates to the root word, we get *under the tongue*. Choice *A*, *in the ear*, would be the word *tympanic*. Choice *B*, in the rectum, would be the word *rectal*. Choice *C*, under the armpit, would be the word *axillary*.

Let's look at a table of popular prefixes.

Prefix	Meaning	Example
ab-	away	abnormality
ad-	at, toward	address
anti-	against	antithesis
auto-	self	autobiography
de-	reverse or change	deduct
dis-	remove	disband
down-	lower	downdraft
ex-	from, out	exacerbate
extra-	beyond	extrapolate
hyper-	extreme	hypertension
il- im- in- ir-	not	illness, impede, indecisive, irregular
inter-	between	interpolate
mid-	middle	midwife
mis-	incorrectly	mistaken
non-	not	nondescript
over-	too much	overwhelmed
out-	go beyond	outer space
poly-	many	polygon
post-	after	postpartum
pre-	before	prefrontal
re-	again	redistribute
sub-	under	sublingual
super-	beyond	superior
trans-	across	transdermal
un-	remove, not	unbearable
under-	less than	underworld
up-	make higher	uppercut

abdomin-	abdomen	abdominal
acou-	hearing	acoustic
adip-	fat	adipose
corono-	heart	coronary
dent-	teeth	dental
dys-	bad, difficult	dysfunction
fract-, frag-	break	fracture
geri-	old age	geriatrics
glyco-	sugar	glycogen
hypo-	below normal	hypotension
iso-	equal	isometric
intra-	within	intravenous
kine-	movement	kinetics
loqu-, locu-	speak	loquacious
mal-	bad, ill	malignant
migr-	move	migratory
myo-	muscle	myocardium
neuro-	nerve	neurologist
omni-	all	omnivorous
pharmac-	medication	pharmaceutical
psych-	mind	psychosomatic
radio-	radiation	radiologist
ren-	kidney	renal
rhino-	nose	rhinovirus
sangui-	blood	sanguine
somn-, somno-	sleep	somnambulant
thermo-	heat	thermometer
toxi-, toxo-	poison	toxoplasmosis
vasculo-	blood vessel	vascular system

Suffix

The word *suffix* is when a **morpheme** (a unit of language) is added at the end of a word. Suffixes are like prefixes, except prefixes go before root words, and suffixes go after root words. One example of a root word with a suffix is the word *accountable*. The word *account* means to consider in a certain way. The suffix *-able* means *capable of being*. If we put the two together, we get *capable of being considered in a certain way*, which is the definition of *accountable*. Let's look at a practice question below:

<u>Question</u>
What is the best definition of the word <u>endogenous</u>?
    a. Characterized by an internal cause
    b. To lift something higher
    c. In a contrary fashion
    d. Not presently active but potentially active

<u>Explanation</u>
Let's look at the word *endogenous* broken down. The suffix *-ous* means *characterized by*. The root word *endogen* means internal or within an organism. Therefore, we have *endogenous*, which means *characterized by internal cause*, Choice A. Choice B, *to lift something higher*, comes from the word *elevate*. Choice C, *in a contrary fashion*, comes from the word *adverse*. Choice D, *not presently active but potentially active*, comes from the word *latent*.

Let's look at a table of popular suffixes:

Suffix	Meaning	Example
-able, -ible	capable of being	debatable
-al	pertaining to	emotional
-esque	similar to	gigantesque
-ful	full of	painful
-ic, -ical	pertaining to	medical
-ious, -ous	characterized by	nutritious, enormous
-ish	having the quality of	childish
-ive	have the nature of	divisive
-less	without	effortless
-y	characterized by	gently
-ate	become	emulate
-en	become	soften
-ify, -fy	make or become	vilify
-ize, -ise	become	socialize
-acy	quality	privacy
-al	act of process of	transdermal
-ance, -ence	state or quality of	dominance
-dom	place or state of being	boredom
-er, -or	one who	doctor
-ism	doctrine, belief	skepticism
-ist	one who	scientist
-ity, -ty, -tude	quality of	activity
-ment, -ness	condition of	settlement
-ship	position held	ownership
-sion, -tion	state of being	comprehension

-algia	pain	fibromyalgia
-asthenia	weak	myasthenia gravis
-cide	killing	fungicide
-coccus	round	streptococcus
-cyte	cell	erythrocyte
-ectomy	removal of	appendectomy
-emia	related to blood	hyperglycemia
-gnosis	knowledge	diagnosis
-itis	Inflammation	tonsillitis
-ology	study of	biology
-oma	tumor	lymphoma
-opsy	examination	autopsy
-ory	related to	auditory
-osis	diseased	osteoporosis
-ostomy, -tomy	surgical cutting	colostomy
-lepsy	seizure	narcolepsy
-pepsia	digestion	dyspepsia
-philia	attracted	hemophilia
-phobia	aversion	claustrophobia
-plegia	paralysis	paraplegia
-pod, -pus	foot	tripod
-pnea	air	sleep apnea
-phyte	grow	zoophyte
-rupt	break	disrupt
-scope	tool used for viewing	stethoscope
-scribe	write	prescribe
-stasis	stopped	homeostasis
-trophy	nourishment	atrophy
-ward	direction	inward

Glossary of Terms

Before going into the exam, it would be helpful to obtain a list of words related to the field of study and memorize them. Many of the words below are root words that have determinable prefixes and suffixes, so test your knowledge by making flash cards and testing your knowledge before you read the definition.

Abstain: to refrain from doing something

Accountable: to be responsible for someone or something

Adhere: to stick or hold together, usually by glue or other bonding material

Adverse: harmful or unfavorable reaction to a medication or situation

Bilateral: relating to or affecting both sides of the body

Concave: a surface that curves inward

Consistency: the thickness or viscosity of something

Constrict: to become smaller or to make narrower

Contraindication: when a situation or procedure may be harmful to the patient because of a certain condition

Defecate: to expel feces from the body

Deficit: a noticeable lack or deficiency in something

Dilute: to make a liquid weaker by adding water to it

Distended: swollen or expanded due to pressure coming from the inside

Elevate: to raise something to a higher position

Endogenous: having been caused by something inside of the body or organism

Exacerbate: to make something worse

Exogenous: to be produced outside the body

Expand: to increase in size or amount

Febrile: having to do with fever

Flaccid: part of the body that hangs limp or loose

Inflamed: redness or swollenness on a part of the body

Insidious: continuing in a gradual way yet with harmful results

Invasive: pertaining to the insertion of medical instruments into the body

Labile: a rapid change that is usually harmful

Latent: to be present but not active or visible

Lethargic: characterized by being sluggish and apathetic

Manifestation: a symptom or sign of an illness that shows up

Occluded: closed or obstructed in some way

Oral: relating or given to by the mouth

Paroxysmal: a sudden or abrupt attack, such as a spasm or a seizure

Precipitous: an action done rapidly and without consideration

Predispose: to make more susceptible or prone to a condition or situation

Preexisting: already existing from an earlier time period

Prognosis: the course or outcome of a particular ailment

Recur: to occur again

Supplement: a product taken that adds to or completes something else

Suppress: to subdue or prevent the expression of something

Symptom: a feature that indicates there is an ailment or disease somewhere present within the body

Grammar

Parts of Speech

Nouns describe people, places, or things. They can represent physical subjects such as *dogs* or *pigs* or intangible things such as *courage* or *spirit.* Nouns can also reflect general things like *man*, but proper nouns address a specific person, place, or thing, like *Howard Marks*.

An **adjective** is a word that modifies the noun itself. Adjectives like *bold*, *brave*, and *big* all provide specific information about the noun being focused on.

Pronouns are sometimes used in place of a noun. For example, one may use *it*, *he*, *she,* and *they* as substitutes for specific people or things.

Verbs represent an action, like *run* and *jump*. They can be in the present, past, and future tense like so: *hike*, *hiked*, and *will hike*.

Sometimes an **adverb** is used to further describe the verb itself. For example, the adverb *quickly* can be used to describe the act of *running*: *he ran quickly.*

Conjunctions are used to join phrases, clauses, and individual words. Conjunctions like *because, or,* and *but* link separate ideas or indicate contrast in order to connect meanings in a sentence. For example: *I like the house, but it's a little large for me.*

Prepositions are inserted before pronouns or nouns to form a phrase; these can include *about, for*, and *with*. Used in a sentence, prepositions work like so: *I decided to write <u>about</u>* The Jungle Book. The preposition creates the phrase: *about* The Jungle Book.

Interjections are words that express strong feelings and are usually accompanied by an exclamation point: *I missed the bus. <u>Oh no!</u>*

Question
Which word from the following sentence is an adjective?

The clever coyote waited until the man wasn't looking to steal the sandwich.

a. coyote
b. waited
c. clever
d. to

Explanation
Choice *C* is the correct answer. *Clever* means quick to understand or learn, so it is describing someone or something, which makes it an adjective. In this case, *clever* is describing *coyote*, which is a noun and the subject of the sentence. Therefore, Choice *A* is incorrect. Choice *B* is incorrect because *waited* is verb, the action of the *coyote*. Choice *D* is incorrect because *to* is a preposition that helps create a phrase that describes the coyote's next action: *to steal the sandwich*.

Sentences

Sentences are created with two core components: the subject and the predicate. The **subject** is the focus of the sentence, someone or something be addressed or talked about. The **predicate** describes the subject. Complete sentences will clearly identify the subject while distinctly indicating the action or information relating to the subject.

A sentence is formed with dependent and independent clauses. A **dependent clause** is a phrase that doesn't make sense on its own but forms a complete sentence when combined with more information. An **independent clause** can stand on its own. They two types of clauses can be combined to form a full sentence like so: _Looking up, I saw that the sun was shining_. Here, with the use of a comma, the dependent clause _Looking up_ is combined with the independent clause _I saw that the sun was shining_ to make a coherent sentence. Sometimes a conjunction and comma are used to combine the clauses.

Proper sentence structure requires subject-verb agreement. Verbs must agree in with the tense and number of the subject(s) for sentences to make sense. As an example: _They is not coming to dinner_. _They_, the subject, is plural while _is_, the verb, is singular. Here's the correction: _They are coming to dinner_.

Select the best word for the blank in the following sentence.

Garth _____ many pets that he cares for.

    a. has
    b. had
    c. have
    d. haves

Explanation

Choice *A* is correct because *has* is the same tense and number as the subject *Garth*, so the verb and subject agree. Choice *B* is incorrect because *had* is past tense while the sentence is clearly present tense, indicated by *that he cares for*. Choice *C* incorrectly uses *have*, which is plural and doesn't agree with the singular subject. Choice *D* is incorrect because *haves* is a plural noun indicating people with possessions, not a verb as is needed here.

Punctuation

Punctuation enables different sections of the sentence to be seamlessly connected so the structure can remain clear while expressing different ideas. Commas are vital for linking independent and dependent clauses to form single sentences. In these cases, commas are usually accompanied by coordinating conjunctions like *but, then, or,* and *and*. See the following example: *I like mushrooms, but I do not like broccoli*. Without a comma to unite dependent and independent clauses, sentences will sound awkward and lack focus. Here's an example: *I bought a cake then I bought ice cream too*.

Without a comma between *cake* and *then*, the sentence seems compressed and disorganized.

Commas can also be used to distinguish items in a list: *run, jump, and ski*. Key points in a sentence can be emphasized through comma use: *After the <u>party, which was at Nick's house, we</u> went to the movies.* Commas are also used to address people directly or direct the readers' attention: *<u>Jim,</u> did you fight a Klingon?* However, there are times when a semicolon is more appropriate to combine two different ideas or independent clauses: *England is a powerful <u>nation; it's been around for centuries.</u>* A writer must use a period (.) after a complete sentence and a question mark (?) for direct questions. Exclamation points (!) are used to emphasize emotion.

Contractions rely on the use of apostrophes—for example, *they are* is reflected in *they're*. An apostrophe with an *s* is also important to remember, for it can be used in a contraction like *it's* (*it is*), or to show possession: *<u>Mike's</u> truck is a Ford*.

<u>Question</u>
Which of the following sentences is grammatically correct?
    a. Hurry its time to see the movie.
    b. Hurry, it's time to see the movie.
    c. Hurry, its time to see the movie.
    d. Hurry; it's time to see the movie

<u>Explanation</u>
Choice *B* is correct because it addresses two glaring punctuational/grammatical issues. First, it adds a comma after *Hurry*, because the speaker is addressing someone directly. The

comma acknowledges this address and transitions into describing why there is need for *hurry*. The second is that *its* is not appropriate for the sentence. *Its* represents the possessive form of *it*, giving it ownership. Instead, what's needed here is the contraction *it's* to indicate that *it is* time to see the movie. Choice *A* is incorrect because it has both issues. Choice *C* applies the comma but uses the possessive *its*. Choice *D* applies the semicolon unnecessarily.

Additional Writing Tips

It's important to be mindful of grammatical rules and sentence structure. The subject should be prominent, while the predicate should be clear and straightforward. A **run-on sentence** is when two independent clauses (complete sentences) are in one sentence but not connected with the proper grammatical structure. Here's an example:

> Tom Brokaw's *The Greatest Generation* is an excellent book on WWII it's a highly recommended book for summer reading.

The way the current sentence is structured doesn't make sense. This sentence should be separated into two sentences or have a semicolon inserted after *WWII*. Alternatively, a comma and coordinating conjunction could be applied to link the two independent clauses.

Another important writing practice is to make sure sentences contain subject-verb agreements. The verb must reflect the same number and tense as the subject in order for the sentence to be coherent, like so: *The cat chases the mouse.* The verb *chases* is singular-present, just like *cat*.

Select the best words for the blanks in the following sentence.

King Richard III is definitely a controversial historical ___ while he is often depicted as a savage tyrant, ___ plenty of evidence to support that he was actually a good king.

  a. figure. However| their are
  b. figure yet, | is
  c. figure as | there be
  d. figure. Yet, | there's

Explanation
Choice *D* is the best answer. The original sentence, as it stands, is a run-on because there needs to be proper punctuation connecting the two independent clauses. Choice *D* is the best answer to correct this because it breaks the sentence into two sentences by putting a period after *figure* and starting a second sentence with *Yet*. By starting with *Yet*, the author is clearly discussing information that shows an alternative viewpoint to the first. *Yet* is also followed by a comma, which is appropriate for introducing/addressing the new information.

The second word, *there's*, is also correct because it is the contraction of *there is*. *There's* is appropriate for indicating the presence of *evidence to support that he was actually a good king*. Choice *A* is tempting. Starting a new sentence with *However* would be a solution, but without a comma following *however*, the sentence will sound jumbled. *Their are* is also incorrect for the sentence, as *their* indicates possession, which is not applicable to the second sentence. Choice *B* is incorrect because it is a run-on. Also, the use of *is* doesn't make sense without the accompanying *there* to modify it. Choice *C* is incorrect for similar reasons—the use of *as* and *be* is grammatically incorrect.

Word Confusion

It's important to be aware that many words have a similar or identical pronunciation, like *affect* and *effect*. *Affect* is a verb, meaning to change or influence something. *Effect*, on the other hand, is a noun reflecting the result or impact of an event or circumstance. Another example is with the verb *see* and the noun *sea*. How the word is used in a particular sentence will indicate which word is needed.

Identifying whether a word is plural, possessive, or a contraction will also eliminate word confusion. For example, *their* shows possession by multiple people, *there* is used to indicate a place or position, and *they're* is a contraction of *they are*. Several spelling variations will give words entirely different meanings. For example, *to* is a preposition indicating motion towards, while the word *too* indicates both *as well as* and *an excessive amount of something* depending on how it's used. The word *two* sounds like *to* and *too*, but it represents the number 2. Memorizing these words and their differences is key. Understanding the context of the sentence as a whole will also reveal which spelling/word is appropriate.

Select the best word for the blank in the following sentence.

Tom couldn't decide which shirt to ___.

a. ware
b. where
c. wear
d. were

Explanation

While all of these words are spelled similarly and sound the same, the correct answer is Choice *C, wear*, which means to cover or equip. We *wear* clothes. Choice *A, ware*, refers to an item that is created or manufactured. Choice *B* is incorrect because *where* asks for a specific location. Choice *D, were*, is the second person plural version of *to be*, so it is completely irrelevant to the sentence.

Biology

Biology Basics

Biology is the study of life and things that are living, including plant and animal species. Organisms are able to survive on their own and have a range of functions, including movement, respiration, growth, and reproduction. All living things are made up of cells. The smallest organisms consist of a single cell, while more complex organisms consist of many different types of cells that function together. Almost all cells contain DNA, which is the genetic material of the organism. DNA is made up of many different genes, each of which is responsible for encoding the traits of the organism. This information is vital for the survival and reproduction of an organism.

There are many different subdisciplines of study within the discipline of biology. Evolution is the study of how organisms change over time. Ecology is the study of how organisms interact with each other and the environment. Genetics is the study of the genes that make up an organism. Botany is the study of plants.

Question
Which subdiscipline of biology would a botanist study?
- a. Growth of an aloe plant
- b. Evolution of monkeys
- c. Genetic changes in human brain cancer
- d. Interaction between worker bees and a queen bee

The correct answer is Choice *A*. Botanists study the field of botany, which is the study of plants. Neither the evolution of monkeys nor the genetic changes in human brain cancer, Choices *B* and *C*, involve studying plants. An ecologist would study how worker bees interact with a queen bee, Choice *D*, because that subdiscipline involves analyzing how organisms interact with each other.

Water

Water has several unique properties. The water molecule is composed of one oxygen atom bonded to two hydrogen atoms, and it forms a V-shape. It is a polar molecule because there is unequal sharing of electrons. Therefore, the oxygen atom remains slightly negative and the hydrogen atoms remain slightly positive. In a solution containing many water molecules, the molecules will bond to each other for a fraction of second when they interact with a weak hydrogen bond.

The figure below shows a water molecule and some of its properties.

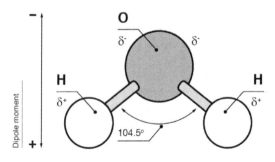

Water is also cohesive and adhesive. **Cohesion** occurs when the same substance bonds to itself. In a glass of water, water molecules can bind to each other at the surface, causing surface tension, which may appear to be a strong film. The surface tension on top of a body of water can keep a raft spider from sinking. **Adhesion** occurs when two different substances link together. Water molecules can bind to the cells in a plant wall to fight gravity, climb the plant, and transport nutrients to the top of the plant.

Question
What shape does a water molecule form?
    a. C-shape
    b. S-shape
    c. V-shape
    d. T-shape

Explanation
The best answer is Choice *C*. Water molecules form a V-shape because of the uneven sharing of electrons between the atoms. The oxygen atom is slightly negatively charged, and the hydrogen atoms are slightly positively charged, so they pull away from each other and the molecule forms a V-shape. As shown in the image, the molecule is in a V-shape and the angle between the two hydrogen atoms is 104.5 degrees.

Biological Molecules

The main elements that comprise biological molecules are carbon, hydrogen, oxygen, nitrogen, sulfur, and phosphorus. Carbon is a common backbone of large molecules because it can bond four different atoms simultaneously. There are four main types of biological molecules: proteins, nucleic acids, lipids, and carbohydrates.

Proteins

Proteins have four levels of structure. The primary structure is the sequence of the amino acids. The secondary structure consists of the folds that are formed by the amino acid chain's backbone binding to itself. The tertiary structure is the overall 3-D shape of the protein caused by folding and side chain binding. The quaternary structure is the overall structure of multiple amino acid chains bound together.

Nucleic Acids

DNA is made up of two strands of nucleotides that bind together and then coil into a helical structure. RNA is made up of a single strand of nucleotides.

Lipids

Lipids are hydrophobic, which means that they do not interact well with water. When water and lipids are mixed together, lipids bind to each other and water binds to itself around the groups of lipids.

Carbohydrates

The simplest carbohydrates, called monosaccharides (such as glucose), are used for cellular respiration. Long-chain carbohydrates, called polysaccharides, which are formed by repeating units of these monosaccharide monomers, can be stored and used for energy at a later time. They also form strong structures when bonded together.

Question
Which type of biological molecule stores information?

    a. Carbohydrates

    b. Nucleic acids

    c. Proteins

    d. Lipids

Explanation
The correct answer is Choice *B*. Nucleic acids include DNA and RNA, which store an organism's genetic information. Carbohydrates, Choice *A*, are used as an energy source for an organism. Proteins, Choice *C*, are important for the structure and function of organisms. Lipids, Choice *D*, are important for energy storage and insulation.

Metabolism

Metabolism is the general term to describe the sum total of the chemical reactions that occur within a cell to synthesize and break down substances. Metabolic reactions often involve an **enzyme**, which is a protein that aids in driving the reaction forward. These reactions can be classified as endergonic or exergonic. **Endergonic reactions** require a source of energy to start the reaction; the products of endergonic reactions contain more free energy than the reactants. **Exergonic reactions** release energy during the reaction; the products of exergonic reactions contain less free energy than the reactants. Cells often use the energy that is released in exergonic reactions as a source of energy for endergonic reactions. This process is called **energy coupling**. Enzymes do not change the overall free energy that drives the reaction but they do make the reaction occur at a faster rate. Enzymes are also designed specifically for certain reactions and cannot work universally for all metabolic reactions.

Question
What changes in a reaction when an enzyme is added?
- a. The amount of free energy stored in the reactants
- b. The number of products that result from the reaction
- c. The amount of free energy stored in the products
- d. The amount of time needed for the reaction to occur

Explanation
The correct answer is Choice *D*. Enzymes increase the rate of the metabolic reaction. They do not change the starting or ending amount of free energy in the reactants or products, so Choices *A* and *C* are incorrect. The number of products also remains the same, so Choice *B* is incorrect.

The Cell

Cells are the smallest unit of living organisms. They provide the basic structure and are the functional unit of all organisms. Organisms can be made up of only one cell or they can be multicellular and comprise many different types of cells together. Prokaryotic cells include bacteria, which are mostly unicellular. Eukaryotic cells include most other animal and plant cells. Organelles are any number of organized structures living inside a cell.

The images on the following pages illustrate a plant cell and an animal cell.

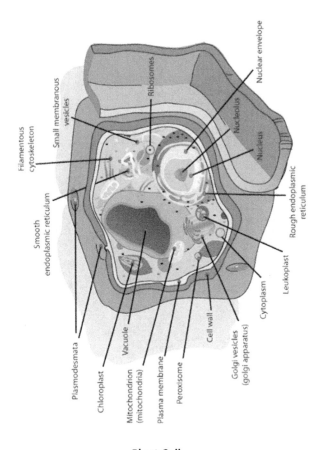

Plant Cell

Nuclear envelope

Ribosomes

Nucleolus

Nucleus

Rough endoplasmic reticulum

Leukoplast

Cytoplasm

Golgi vesicles (golgi apparatus)

Cell wall

Peroxisome

Plasma membrane

Mitochondrion (mitochondria)

Vacuole

Chloroplast

Plasmodesmata

Smooth endoplasmic reticulum

Filamentous cytoskeleton

Small membranous vesicles

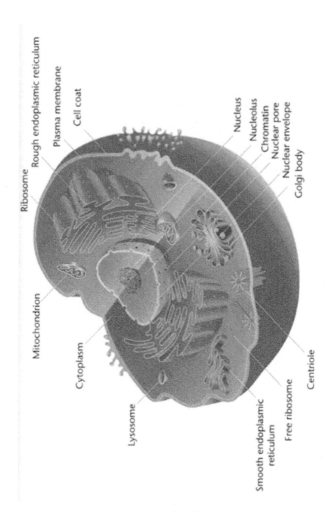

Animal Cell

If a molecule were trying to enter an animal cell, which organelle would it have to pass through first?

    a. Cell wall

    b. Cell membrane

    c. Nucleus

    d. Endoplasmic reticulum

Explanation

The correct answer is Choice *B*. An animal cell is surrounded by a cell membrane. The cell membrane contains proteins that regulate which molecules are allowed in and out of the cell. Only plant cells are surrounded by a cell wall, so Choice *A* is incorrect. The nucleus, Choice *C*, is located in middle of the cell and would not be the first organelle that a molecule would encounter. The endoplasmic reticulum, Choice *D*, is located within the cytoplasm, inside the cell membrane.

Cellular Respiration

Cellular respiration occurs when a cell converts energy from nutrients into adenosine triphosphate (ATP). If the metabolic reaction uses oxygen, it is called **aerobic respiration**, and if it occurs without using oxygen, it is called **anaerobic respiration**. Aerobic respiration begins with glycolysis, which is the conversion of glucose (a common molecule used to generate energy) into pyruvate. Then, pyruvate enters the citric acid cycle and once that is completed, the products go through oxidative phosphorylation. The citric acid cycle generates four ATP molecules. The oxidative phosphorylation process generates 26 to 28 ATP molecules. In total, aerobic respiration generates 30 to 32 ATP molecules that can be used to drive other metabolic reactions forward. Organisms that live in oxygen-poor environments can use anaerobic respiration to generate ATP molecules for energy. The process is less efficient and generates fewer ATP molecules than aerobic respiration, but it is a viable alternative for organisms that do not have oxygen readily available.

Question

Which of the following represents a possible number of ATP molecules for oxidative phosphorylation to generate?

    a. 26

    b. 30

    c. 4

    d. 36

Explanation

The correct answer is Choice *A*. Oxidative phosphorylation is the final part of aerobic respiration and generates between 26 and 28 ATP molecules. In total, aerobic respiration generates between 30 and 32 ATP molecules, Choice *B*. Glycolysis and the citric acid cycle are the first parts of aerobic respiration and generate four ATP molecules, Choice *C*.

Photosynthesis

Photosynthesis is the process by which plants convert light energy into chemical energy. The chemical energy can be used right away or stored as sugar for use at a later time. The process takes place inside the chloroplasts in the plant cells. Photosynthesis has two distinct stages: the light reactions and the Calvin cycle. During the light reactions, light energy gets absorbed by the chlorophyll molecules inside the chloroplasts.

Photons from the light pass through many electron transporting reactions and eventually ATP and NADPH (nicotinamide adenine dinucleotide phosphate) molecules, both forms of energy, are produced. These are passed on to the Calvin cycle. During the Calvin cycle, carbon dioxide from the air is absorbed by the chloroplasts. Another series of reactions occurs, and a sugar molecule is produced at the end of the photosynthetic process. For every sugar molecule that is produced, nine ATP molecules and six NADPH molecules are consumed.

The figure below shows the basic chemical reaction of photosynthesis.

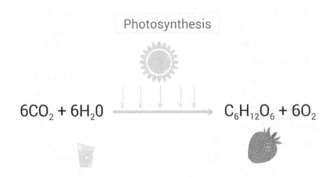

Photosynthesis

$$6CO_2 + 6H_2O \longrightarrow C_6H_{12}O_6 + 6O_2$$

Question

Which is a product of the photosynthetic reaction, as shown in the figure above?

    a. CO_2

    b. H_2O

    c. O_2

    d. Solar energy

The correct answer is Choice *C*. As on the right side of the chemical equation in the image, O_2 is one of the products of the reaction. The left side of the equation contains the reactants. The reactants are CO_2, which is Choice *A*, and H_2O, which is Choice *B*. Solar energy, Choice *D*, joins the reactants to drive the reaction forward.

Cellular Reproduction

The process by which cells replicate and divide into new cells is called **cellular reproduction**. This process allows multicellular organisms to replenish dead and dying cells, and it is a crucial part of maintaining viability. Cells can divide by mitosis, which creates an identical daughter cell, or by meiosis, which creates a daughter cell with similarities to each parent cell without being identical to either one. Division by mitosis has five steps: prophase, prometaphase, metaphase, anaphase, and telophase. The chromosomes of one cell replicate, and then the entire cell divides into two separate cells in a stage called cytokinesis. Meiosis involves two sets of division. Two non-identical parent cells combine, and their chromosomes replicate and mix with each other, creating four new chromosomes that are not identical to each other or to the original parents. This cell then goes through two sets of mitosis steps and ends with four daughter cells.

The table below describes similarities and differences between mitosis and meiosis.

Property	Mitosis	Meiosis
DNA Replication	Occurs during interphase before the start of mitosis.	Occurs during interphase before the start of meiosis.
Number of Divisions	One	Two
Synapsis of Homologous Chromosomes	Does not occur in mitosis.	Occurs with crossing over between non-sister chromatids in prophase I.
Number of Daughter Cells and Genetic Composition	Two diploid (2n) daughter cells genetically identical to parent cell are produced.	Four haploid (n) daughter cells that contain half as many chromosomes as the parent cell. Daughter cells are genetically different from each other as well as the parent cell.
Role in Animal Body	Produces cells for growth and repair.	Produces gametes and maintains genetic diversity in sexual reproduction.

<u>Question</u>

Which of the following is identical in both mitosis and meiosis?

    a. The number of divisions

    b. The number of daughter cells produced

    c. The synapsis of homologous chromosomes

    d. When DNA replication occurs

<u>Explanation</u>

The correct answer is Choice *D*. In both mitosis and meiosis, DNA replication occurs during interphase. Mitosis has one cell division whereas meiosis has two cell divisions; therefore, Choice *A*, the number of divisions, is incorrect. Mitosis produces two daughter cells whereas meiosis produces four daughter cells; therefore, Choice *B* is incorrect. Synapsis of homologous chromosomes, Choice *C*, does not occur in mitosis.

Genetics

Genetics is the study of traits and how they are passed down between generations. Gregor Mendel, a scientist and 19th-century monk, is considered the father of genetics. In the 1860s, he developed one of the first models of heredity and inheritance, based on his research with pea pod plants and the colors of their flowers. He came up with three laws that can still be applied to genetics today.

1. The law of dominance: If a trait is dominant, that phenotype will always be seen in future generations. It will always mask the recessive trait if it is present.

2. The law of segregation: Each parent has two alleles of each gene. During meiosis, the two alleles will be separated from each other. They are not linked together.

3. The law of independent assortment: Inheritance of every gene during the second division of meiosis is independent of all other genes. Even if genes reside on the same chromosome, the alleles of each gene are randomly sorted and assigned.

Question

Which of Mendel's laws of inheritance states that a dominant phenotype will always be seen over a recessive phenotype?

    a. The law of dominance
    b. The law of similarity
    c. The law of segregation
    d. The law of independent assortment

Explanation

The correct choice is Choice *A*. The law of dominance states that dominant traits are always passed on and will be present in future generations, even if recessive alleles are inherited. Choice *B*, the law of similarity, is not one of Mendel's laws. The law of segregation, Choice *C*, states that the alleles of a gene are separated during meiosis. The law of independent assortment, Choice *D*, states that genes on the same chromosome are all independently and randomly sorted and assigned during the second division of meiosis.

DNA

DNA contains the genetic material of an organism. It consists of two polynucleotide strands that are linked together and twisted to form a double-helix structure. There are four nitrogenous bases that make up DNA: adenine, thymine, guanine, and cytosine. These bases pair with each other in specific ways. Adenine and thymine always pair together, while guanine and cytosine always pair together. Adenine and guanine are purines, whereas thymine and cytosine are pyrimidines. The bases have different base structures. When DNA replicates, the two polynucleotide strands are untwisted and separated, and then a new pairing strand is generated for each of the separated strands. When the replication process is finished, each new DNA molecule contains one original strand and one newly replicated strand.

The figure below shows the difference in structure between purines and pyrimidines.

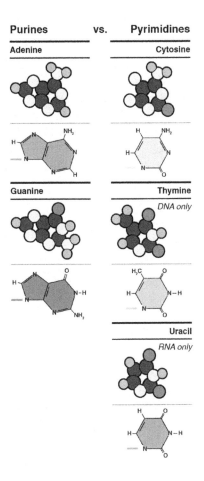

Which base pairs up with adenine in DNA?

    a. Uracil

    b. Thymine

    c. Guanine

    d. Cytosine

Explanation

The correct answer is Choice *B*. In DNA, adenine pairs only with thymine. Uracil, Choice *A*, is only found in RNA, not DNA. Guanine and cytosine, Choices *C* and *D*, pair with each other exclusively in DNA.

Chemistry

Scientific Notation, the Metric System, and Temperature Scales

Scientific notation is useful for expressing very small or large quantities. Scientific notation represents a number in the form $A \times 10^n$, where A is a nonzero digit (one–nine) to the left of the decimal point and n is a positive or negative whole number. For example, the Empire State Building in New York stands 1454 feet (ft) tall, and, in scientific notation, this would equate to 1.454×10^3 ft, precise to four significant figures. The speed of light is 6.71×10^8 miles per hour (mph), or 670,616,629 mph.

The international system of units (SI) is a specific choice of metric units that consists of SI base units and an SI prefix. The SI base units describe quantities such as length and mass, which have units of a meter (m) and kilogram (kg). For example, one foot or twelve inches is equal to 0.3048 meters, where meters is an SI base unit that describes the length in the metric system. An SI prefix designates powers of ten and describes relatively large or small quantities. The SI prefix that uses the multiple 10^{-2} meters (or 0.01 m) is equal to one centimeter (cm). Other SI prefixes include micro (μ)-(10^{-6}), milli (m)- (10^{-3}), kilo (k)- (10^3), and mega(M)-(10^6), to name a few. Other SI base quantities include the second (s), which is a unit of time.

Temperature is another SI base quantity with units of Kelvin (K), which is an absolute scale where the temperature can be theoretically zero. The temperature measures the "hotness" of a substance. The scientific community commonly uses another temperature scale called the Celsius (°C) scale. In contrast, the United States uses the Fahrenheit (°F) scale. The following equations show how to convert from one scale to another.

$$1. T_C = \frac{5°C}{9°F} \times (T_F - 32°F)$$

$$2. T_k = 273.15K + \left(T_C \times \frac{1\,K}{1°C}\right)$$

Question
In the United States, the average temperature for water coming out of a hot spring is 143°F. What is the average temperature for a hot spring in Celsius and Kelvin? Express the final answer in milliKelvin (mK) and then convert to scientific notation.

    a. 334,800 μ K and 3.348 $\times 10^6$ μK
    b. 334,800 mK and 3.348 $\times 10^{-6}$ mK
    c. 334,800 mK and 3348 $\times 10^2$ mK
    d. 334,800 mK and 3.348 $\times 10^6$ mK

Explanation
The correct answer choice is Choice *D*, which expresses the answer in mK and scientific notation. The first step is to convert °F to °C using Equation 1.

$$T_C = \frac{5°C}{9°F} \times \left(14\underline{3}°F - 32°F\right) = \frac{5°C}{9°F}\left(11\underline{1}°F\right) = \mathbf{61.\underline{7}°C}$$

The answer is rounded and precise to three significant figures, giving 61.7°C. Use the unrounded answer when performing subsequent calculations.

The next step is to convert Celsius (°C) to Kelvin (K).

$$T_k = 273.15\ K + \left(61.\overline{6}\,°C \times \frac{1\ K}{1°C}\right) = \boldsymbol{334.8\ K}$$

The previous answer ($61.\overline{6}\,°C$) has three significant figures. The °C units cancel out within the brackets. When adding, the addition/subtraction rules for significant figures must be followed. because $61.\overline{6}\,°C$ has one significant figure after the decimal point, the final answer (rounded) is 334.8 K. Converting this answer to scientific notation (precise to four significant figures) gives:

$$334.8\ K = 3.348 \times 10^2\ K$$

The multiple for the prefix *milli-* (m) is 10^{-3}. It is essential to set up the expression correctly when converting to different units. When converting from a large to a small quantity (e.g., K to mK), then 1 K = 10^3 mK ($10^3\ mK = 1000\ K = 1.\times 10^3\ K$). When converting from a small to a large quantity (e.g., mK to K), then 1 mK = 10^{-3} K ($10^{-3}\ K = 0.001\ K = 1.\times 10^{-3}\ K$). The conversions below show conversion from K to mK and mK to K:

K to mK (large answer):

$$334.8\ K \times \left(\frac{10^3\ mK}{1\ K}\right) = 334{,}800\ mK$$

mK to K (small answer):

$$334{,}800 \ mK \times \left(\frac{10^{-3} \ K}{1 \ mK}\right) = 334.8 \ K$$

In scientific notation, 334,800 mK equals $3.348 \times 10^6 \ mK$, which is precise to four significant figures. However, expressing the answer in units of Kelvin (334.8 K) is simple, which demonstrates the reason why a prefix (or scientific notation) may not be necessary for this problem. Answer Choice C is numerically correct ($3348 \times 10^2 \ mK$), but does not follow the correct scientific format (A is a number between 1–9 before the decimal point).

Atomic Structure and the Periodic Table

The nuclear model describes the atom having a dense center of positive charge (the nucleus) with electrons moving around the center at a distance much greater than the nuclear radius. The size of the nucleus to an atom is like a small marble to the size of a football stadium, indicating that the atom is mostly space. The nucleus contains a positively-charged proton and a neutrally-charged neutron, which both have roughly the same mass. The mass of an electron is around 1800 times less than the mass of the proton or neutron.

In 1869, both Dmitri Mendeleev and Julius Meyer published the present form of the periodic table. Based on specific properties of other elements within a group, Mendeleev showed how the table could be used to predict the properties of new elements. An **element** is identified by an atomic number (Z) that indicates the total amount of protons. Because an element is neutral in charge, the number of electrons must equal to Z. Some periodic tables show a mass number (A), a whole number, that is equal to the sum of all neutrons and protons.

The current periodic table orders the elements based on atomic number, which increases across the period or row and down a column or group. The specific arrangement of elements in the periodic table has several emerging trends that allow for a qualitative prediction of periodic properties such as atomic radius and electron affinity. For instance, within a group, the **atomic radius** of an atom increases from top to bottom (e.g., Li to Cs) because the number of electrons or principal quantum number (n =1, 2, 3, etc.) increases. The atomic radius decreases along the period or row from left to right, due to an effective nuclear charge (more protons pull valence electrons inward).

Metals, nonmetals, and metalloid elements make up the periodic table. Groups 1A and 2A consist primary of metals, and groups 7A and 8A consist of nonmetals. The charge on an element can be predicted using a periodic table. For metals found in the first two columns of the periodic table, the charge of the ion is equal to the group number. Sodium is in group 1A, so it will lose one electron to form Na^+. Nonmetals, such as the halogens, tend to gain an electron with a charge equal to eight minus its group number. For main group elements (Groups 1–8A), the group number is also equal to the number of valence electrons.

Using your knowledge of the period table, which of the following make logical sense in terms of the charges on F and Mg?

    a. F^{-8} (8-); Mg^{1+} (!+)
    b. F^{-7} (7-); Mg^{2+} (2+)
    c. F^- (1-); Mg^{1+} (1+)
    d. F^- (1-); Mg^{2+} (2+)

Explanation

The correct answer choice is Choice *D*. Fluorine (F), a halogen, is a nonmetal found in Group 7A. The F atom will accept one electron to form a 1- charge. The number is written before the sign and placed on the superscript to indicate charge. This charge is written as a superscript on the right-hand side (1-) without the number because the charge is one, F^- (fluoride ion). The atomic number for F is nine, so there must be nine electrons for the atom to be neutral. When the F element accepts one electron to form F^-, there will be ten electrons. Fluoride(F^-) will have the same number of electrons as neon (Ne).

Magnesium (Mg) is an alkaline earth metal found in Group 2A. The Mg atom will lose two electrons to form a 2+ charge. This charge is shown as a superscript on the right-hand side (2+): Mg^{2+} with the number before the sign. The atomic number for the Mg element is twelve, so there will be twelve electrons. However, Mg will lose two electrons to form the Mg^{2+} ion, which has ten electrons. The Mg^{2+} ion will have the same number of electrons as neon (Ne).

Ions like F^- or Mg^{2+} form stable noble gas configurations like Ne gas.

Chemical Equations

A chemical equation is the symbolic representation of a molecular reaction using chemical formulas, phase labels, reaction arrows, and coefficients. Consider the reaction of chlorine gas (Cl_2) with potassium (K), which involves the rearrangement of the potassium and chlorine (Cl) atoms to yield a new combination of atoms in potassium chloride (KCl). The reaction equation shows the production of potassium chloride:

$$2K(s) + Cl_2(g) \rightarrow 2KCl(s)$$

The chemical formulas, K and Cl_2 on the left-hand side of the reaction equation (before the arrow $\rightarrow$), are called the **reactants.** The formula KCl, on the right side of the reaction equation (after the $\rightarrow$), represents the created product or substance. On the reactant side, the "+" means that the reactants are combining. The arrow ($\rightarrow$) means "react to form" or "produced." The coefficients in the equation show the number of molecules or formula units (e.g., KCl). The mass of two potassium atoms and one chlorine molecule must be equal to the total mass of two potassium chloride units, which is consistent with the *law of conservation of mass*. Coefficients are typically placed in front of the chemical formula to ensure that the equation is balanced such that the masses of each side are equal. Coefficients of "1" are not shown, and these numbers are not to be confused with subscripts or superscripts. For example, the equation says that two molecules of solid potassium (K) react with one molecule of chlorine gas (Cl_2) to produce two molecules of solid potassium chloride (KCl). The states of the substances are placed to the right of the chemical formula and are indicated in parentheses by the following labels: (s) = solid, (l) = liquid, (g) = gas, and (aq) = aqueous water solution. Sometimes, symbols are placed over the reaction arrows to indicate the reaction occurs under heat ($\xrightarrow{\Delta}$) or with a catalyst such as platinum ($\xrightarrow{Pt}$). The reaction of K and Cl_2 is an example of a **combination reaction** because two components combine to form one single component, KCl. The opposite is a **decomposition reaction**, such as that where $Cu(OH)_2$ produces two products, copper oxide (CuO) and water:

$$Cu(OH)_2(s) \rightarrow CuO\ (s) + H_2O(g)$$

Another type is the **double replacement (displacement)** reaction, such as that between sodium hydroxide (NaOH, shampoo) and hydrochloric acid (HCl, stomach acid), which produces water and sodium chloride (NaCl, table salt).

$$NaOH\ (aq) + HCl(aq) \rightarrow H_2O(l) + NaCl(aq)$$

In the **acid-base reaction**, OH and Cl exchange places, as do Na and H. In **single-replacement (displacement) reactions,** the exchange occurs between one pair of species. For example, in the oxidation-reduction reaction of zinc (Zn) with silver nitrate ($AgNO_3$), Zn and Ag exchange places to produce silver (Ag) and $ZnNO_3$.

$$Zn\ (s) + 2AgNO_3(aq) \rightarrow 2Ag(s) + Zn(NO_3)_2(aq)$$

Some compounds, such as copper (II) hydroxide ($Cu(OH)_2$), the blue pigment used in old paintings (e.g., Maya paintings of Calakmul), decompose to a black product, which is responsible for the degradation of many Renaissance paintings.

Question

In an industrial reaction called the Haber process, the reaction of hydrogen (H_2) and nitrogen (N_2) gas with an iron (Fe) catalyst, at high pressure and temperatures, yields ammonia gas (NH_3). Which of the following correctly shows the complete balanced equation for this reaction?

a. $H + N_2 \xrightarrow{Fe} NH_3$

b. $3H + N_2 \xrightarrow{Fe} NH_3$

c. $3H_2 + N_2 \xrightarrow{Fe} 2NH_3$

d. $3H_2 + N_2 \xrightarrow{Fe} 3NH_3$

Explanation

Choice *C* is the correct answer. In a chemical reaction, the products are the produced substances; in this case, ammonia gas (NH_3) is the product. The reactants are hydrogen (H_2) and nitrogen gas (N_2). The chemical equation must be balanced by placing the appropriate coefficients for each chemical formula. For example, on the left side, there is one molecule of H_2, which contains two bonded H atoms. H has an atomic mass unit (amu) of 1.00794 amu, so the total mass is 2×1.00794 amu. On the right side, there are three H atoms bonded to one N atom. The mass of hydrogen is 3×1.00794 amu. The least common factor of two and three is six, meaning there must be six H atoms on each side of the equation. The equation can be balanced by placing a coefficient of 3 in front of H_2 and 2 in front of NH_3.

$$3H_2(g) + N_2(g) \xrightarrow{Fe} 2NH_3(g)$$

By placing the indicated coefficients in front of H_2 and NH_3, the number of N atoms is also balanced on each side. Alternatively, the nitrogen atoms could have been balanced first by placing a coefficient of 2 in front of NH_3, which would indicate that a 3 would have to be placed in front of H_2.

The molecular interpretation is that three molecules of hydrogen gas (H_2) react with one molecule of nitrogen gas (N_2) to produce two molecules of ammonia gas (NH_3). Nitrogen has a molecular mass of 14.00674 amu. The mass interpretation says that $3 \times 2.01588 \; grams \; (g)$ of hydrogen gas (H_2) reacts with 28.01348 g of nitrogen gas (N_2) to produce $2 \times 17.03056 \; g$ of ammonia gas (NH_3). The sum of the masses on both sides of the equation are equal to 34.1 g, precise to three significant figures.

Reaction Rates, Equilibrium, and Reversibility

The rate of a chemical reaction, or **reaction rate**, indicates how much reactant is consumed or the amount of product that is formed per unit of time. For a specific reaction, the rate of product formation can be increased or decreased by controlling variables such as pressure, temperature, and the concentration of reactants or catalysts. The production of ammonia through the Haber process makes use of an iron (Fe) catalyst and a metal oxide to speed up the reaction:

$$3H_2(g) + N_2(g) \rightarrow 2NH_3(g)$$

The production of ammonia is exothermic and releases heat in the forward direction. Based on Le Chatelier's principle, increasing the temperature would make the forward reaction less favorable ($K \sim 1$ at $200°C$ and $K = 4 \times 10^{-3}$ at $300°C$). To increase the reaction rate, pressures up to 200 atmospheric units can be applied to push the reaction forward. Based on Le Chatelier's principle, pressure favors the products, as two moles of NH_3 are formed compared to four moles of reactant. The rate is expressed as the decrease or increase in molar concentration of the reactant or product per unit time. The units of the reaction rate are moles per liter second ($moles \times Liter^{-1} \times second^{-1}$ or $mol/(L \times s)$).

The average reaction rate can be expressed in three different ways:

$$Rate\ of\ formation\ of\ ammonia = \frac{\Delta[NH_3]}{\Delta t}$$

$$Rate\ of\ decomposition\ of\ nitrogen = -\frac{\Delta[N_2]}{\Delta t}$$

$$Rate\ of\ decomposition\ of\ hydrogen = -\frac{\Delta[H_2]}{\Delta t}$$

The triangle "Δ" signals a change in the reaction rates (not heat) and the enclosed brackets denote the molar concentration or molarity (M, mol/L) of the substance. The reaction rate expressed regarding ammonia gas can be read as: the rate of formation of NH_3 is equal to the change in molar concentration of ammonia gas over the change in time. For the reactants, N_2 and H_2, there is a minus sign ($-$) placed in front because these concentrations decrease over time. Initially, the rate of formation or decomposition will be relatively high but will decrease over time until the reaction rate is constant. The reaction approaches a dynamic chemical equilibrium when the rate of formation or decomposition progress at an equal rate.

Chemical equilibrium does not mean that the concentrations for the reactants and products will be equal. At dynamic equilibrium, there will be a specific ratio or exchange of products to reactants, and no net change will occur. In contrast, a chemical reaction at static equilibrium will have no exchange because it proceeds irreversibly from reactants → products with a reaction rate of zero in either (forward/reverse) direction. The conversion of diamond to graphite (pencil tip) at room temperature is one example. The expressions for the forward and reverse rates are equivalent when incorporating the coefficients from the balanced equation. For instance, the rate of formation of N_2 is twice as fast as the rate of decomposition of NH_3, which is shown by dividing the coefficient 1 of N_2 over the coefficient of 2 from NH_3: $(1/2) \times rate\ of\ N_2\ decomposition = rate\ of\ NH_3\ formation$. The reaction is reversible, as a small change in a condition (temperature, pressure) can make the process go either in the reverse or forward direction. The reversible reaction or dynamic equilibrium for the production of ammonia is indicated by the forward and reverse arrows:

$$3H_2(g) + N_2(g) \rightarrow 2NH_3(g)$$

What will happen if the pressure in the following system is increased after equilibrium was achieved?

$$3O_2(g) \rightleftarrows 2O_3(g)$$

a. There will be no change unless temperature is increased as well.

b. There will be no change unless temperature is decreased as well.

c. More O_3 will be formed (reaction rate will increase in the forward direction).

d. More O_2 will be formed (reaction rate will increase in the reverse direction).

Explanation

Choice C is correct. Based on La Chatelier's Principle, in gaseous reactions, when pressure is increased, volume decreases; thus, the reaction favors the side of the equation with fewer moles of gas. The "product" side of the equation, in this case, has two moles of gas versus three in the "reactant" side. (Because this reaction is reversible, it could have been written either way.) Therefore, when pressure is increased, the reaction will shift to making more of the O_3.

Solutions and Solution Concentrations

Most substances, such as shampoos, coffee, and gasoline, exist as mixtures. A solution contains components of the mixture that are mixed uniformly or **homogeneous.** These solutions may exist as solids, liquids, and gases. For example, seawater contains a solid salt mixture (e.g., NaCl) dissolved in liquid water. The salt is called the **solute** because it is the smaller component, and liquid water is called the **solvent** because it is the large component in the solution. Therefore, a solution is composed of a solute and a solvent. Air is an example of a gaseous solution where nitrogen gas (seventy-eight percent by volume) is considered the solvent, and oxygen (twenty-one percent) and argon (0.93 percent) are the solute components. If the solution is **dilute,** there is relatively little solute, and if the solution is **concentrated,** there is relatively more solute. Solution composition can be described by concentration or **molarity** *(M),* which is the number of moles of solute over a liter of solution (moles/ Liter or mol/L). Solution composition can be described by **mass percent**, which is the percent solute by mass within the solution:

$$Mass \% = \left(\frac{Grams\ of\ solute\ (g)}{Grams\ of\ solution\ (g)} \right) \times 100\%$$

Mole fraction *(χ)*is equal to the number of moles (n) of one substance divided by the total number of moles for all substances in the solution. The solution contains the solute and solvent. For example, assuming a two-component system, the mole fraction of salt in seawater may be represented as:

$$Mole\ fraction\ of\ salt = \chi_{salt} = \frac{n_{salt}}{n_{salt} + n_{seawater}}$$

Molality *(m)* is another way of expressing concentration and is the number of moles of solute divided by kilograms of solvent (mol/kg):

$$Molality = \chi_{salt} = \frac{Moles\ of\ solute}{Kilograms\ of\ solvent}$$

Question

A smooth sweet tea recipe calls for 150 grams of glucose ($C_6H_{12}O_6$) and 1400 grams of water. What is the molarity of this mixture? (Use the following molar masses for C, H, O: C=12.01 g/mol, H=1.008 g/mol, and O=16.0 g/mol. The density of water is 1 g/mL.)

a. $M = 0.695\ mol/L$
b. $M = 0.595\ mol/L$
c. $M = 0.505\ mol/L$
d. $M = 0.650\ mol/L$

Explanation

Choice *B* is the correct answer. To find the molarity, first find the molar mass of glucose, which is about 180.2 grams/mole because $(6 \times 12.01\ amu) + (12 \times 1.008\ amu) + (6 \times 16.0\ amu) = 180.2$ amu or grams/mole. The number of moles of glucose is calculated by dividing the mass of glucose over the molar mass of glucose. Applying dimensional analysis gives g/(g/mol) $= g \cdot g^{-1} \cdot mol = moles$. The mass of water is converted to liters of solution given that the density of water is 1 gram/milliliter. The expression for molarity is:

$$Molarity = \frac{Moles\ of\ solute}{Liters\ of\ solution}$$

$$= \frac{150\ Grams\ \text{glucose} \times \left(\frac{1\ Mole\ glucose}{180.2\ (Grams \cdot mole^{-1})\ glucose}\right)}{1400\ Grams\ of\ water\ \times \left(\frac{1\ mL\ Water}{1\ Gram\ water}\right) \times \left(\frac{1\ L\ Water}{1000\ mL\ Water}\right)}$$

$= 0.595\ M$ (to three significant figures).

Chemical Reactions

A common chemical reaction that occurs in an aqueous solution is a **precipitate reaction**, which occurs when a cation and an anion combine to form an insoluble solid ionic substance. In solution, a precipitate may be evident by a color change or cloudy-colored solution. Substances that break apart in water are called **electrolytes,** which create an electrically-conducting solution. For example, sodium chloride (NaCl) or table salt is an electrolyte. Table salt (NaCl) dissolves in liquid water to form a sodium (Na^+) cation and a chloride (Cl^-) anion.

$$NaCl(s) \xrightarrow{H_2O} Na^+(aq) + Cl^-(aq)$$

Sodium chloride is a strong electrolyte because the solution is composed mostly of ions. Some substances, such as sugar or glucose ($C_6H_{12}O_6$), are nonelectrolytes or poorly conducting solutions because the molecule does not break apart when dissolved in water.

$$C_6H_{12}O_6(s) \xrightarrow{H_2O} C_6H_{12}O_6(aq)$$

The sugar molecule does not decompose into charged parts like sodium chloride. Sugar and sodium chloride are both soluble in water. Some compounds are not soluble and form a precipitate, which occurs when two different electrolyte solutions are mixed. For example, consider the **exchange** or **metathesis reaction** of potassium iodide (KI, Solution 1) and lead (II) nitrate ($Pb(NO_3)_2$, Solution 2), which forms a precipitate called lead (II) iodide (PbI_2).

The complete molecular equation shows one precipitate:

$$2\,KI(aq) + Pb(NO_3)_2\,(aq) \rightarrow 2\,KNO_3(aq) + PbI_2(s)$$

Both reactants and products are written as molecular substances; however, because the reactants are strong electrolytes, they will dissolve completely and exist as ions. In the exchange reaction, there is an exchange of parts between the two reactants. When the lead (II) ion (Pb^{2+}) combines with nitrate (NO_3^-), the ionic compound becomes insoluble and forms a precipitate in solution. The table below is useful for predicting whether an ionic compound, formed when mixing two electrolyte solutions, will be soluble or insoluble.

Ionic Salt	Solubility	Exceptions
Group I element-containing salts and NH_4^+-containing salts	Soluble	None
Nitrites and acetates (NO_3^- and $C_2H_3O_2^-$)	Soluble	None
Cl^-, Br^-, or I^- containing salts	Soluble	Halide salts of Ag^+, Pb^{2+}, and $(Hg_2)^{2+}$
Sulfate salts (SO_4^{2-})	Soluble	Group 2A compounds: $CaSO_4$, $BaSO_4$, $PbSO_4$, Ag_2SO_4 and $SrSO_4$
Silver salts	Insoluble	$AgNO_3$ and $Ag(C_2H_3O_2)$
Hydroxide salts (OH^-) of Group I elements	Soluble	
Hydroxide salts (OH^-) of Group II elements	Slightly soluble	
Hydroxide salts (OH^-) and sulfides (S^{2-}) of transition metals and Al^{3+}	Insoluble	
Silver salts	Insoluble	$AgNO_3$ and $Ag(C_2H_3O_2)$
Carbonates (CO_3^{2-}), Chromates, Phosphates (PO_4^{3-}), and Fluorides (F^-)	Insoluble	

Question

A precipitate reaction forms which of the following?

    a. An insoluble salt

    b. A soluble salt

    c. A cation

    d. An anion

Choice *A* is the correct answer. In a precipitation reaction, solutions that contain a cation and an anion combine to form an insoluble solid ionic substance. This insoluble solid is called a precipitate, which is how the reaction type's name was derived. Choice *B* is incorrect because if the product formed was soluble, it would be dissolved rather than form a visible precipitate. Choices *C* and *D* are incorrect. Neither a cation nor anion, specifically, are *formed* in a precipitation reaction. Rather, the aqueous solutions that are combined in a precipitation reaction each contain either a cation or anion. It is the cation/anion pair in the resulting combined solution (from the reactants of the anion in solution and cation in solution) that forms the precipitate

Stoichiometry

In a chemical reaction, **stoichiometry** is the study of the quantities of materials consumed (reactants) and produced (products). When performing chemical calculations that involve quantities, one must understand the concept of a **mole** *(mol)* and how it relates to the mass of a substance. The mole is a unit for an amount of substance and is equal to the number of carbon atoms in twelve grams of carbon-12. One mole of any substance is equal to 6.022×10^{23} (Avogadro's number) units of that substance. Each element in the periodic table has a unique atomic mass, expressed in grams, and contains one mole of atoms. For every 1.008 grams of hydrogen (H), there is one mole of hydrogen atoms. For example, consider the scenario where one nectarine has a mass of 0.250 grams, and one grapefruit has a mass of 1.0 gram. If the fruits were placed in separate containers (mole), the container holding grapefruit would be four times heavier than the one containing nectarines, but both containers will have the same number of fruit. This idea extends to elements and molecular compounds. For example, one mole of the C element contains 6.022×10^{23} C atoms, and for every one mole of C there are 12.01 grams of C. One mole of water contains 6.022×10^{23} water molecules, and for every one mole of water, there are 18.0 grams of water. Consider the following reaction:

$$3H_2(g) + N_2(g) \rightarrow 2NH_3(g)$$

The equation describes how three molecules of hydrogen gas react with one molecule of nitrogen gas. A similar statement involving multiples of the molecules incorporates Avogadro's number: $3 \times (6.022 \times 10^{23}\ molecules)$ of hydrogen gas combine with $1 \times (6.022 \times 10^{23}\ molecules)$ of nitrogen gas to produce $2 \times (6.022 \times 10^{23}\ molecules)$ of ammonia gas. Because one mole is equal to $6.022 \times 10^{23}\ molecules$, the molar interpretation can be stated as 3 moles H_2 + 1 moles N_2 $\rightarrow$ 2 moles NH_3. The stoichiometric relationship in the chemical equation allows the mass conversion of H2 to the mass of N_2 or NH_3. Consider the following examples:

1. Converting moles of H_2 to moles of N_2 using a unit type conversion with the fixed stoichiometric ratio (1 mole N_2 = 3 moles of H_2) from the balanced equation. The amount 2.0 moles H_2 is arbitrary:

$$2.0\ Moles\ H_2 \times \left(\frac{1\ Mole\ N_2}{3\ Moles\ H_2} \right) = 6.0\ Moles\ N_2$$

2. Converting moles of H_2 to moles of NH_3 using the fixed stoichiometric ratio (3 moles H_2 = 2 moles of NH_3) from the balanced equation:

$$2.0 \: Moles \: H_2 \times \left(\frac{2 \: Moles \: NH_3}{3 \: Moles \: H_2}\right) = 1.3 \: Moles \: NH_3$$

Question
In the reaction below, if 500 grams of hydrogen reacted with excess nitrogen, what is the mass of produced ammonia gas in the reaction? Use the following molar masses, if needed: N_2 = 28.0 g/mol, H_2 = 2.02 g/mol, and NH_3 = 17.0 g/mol.

$$3H_2(g) + N_2(g) \rightarrow 2NH_3(g)$$

a. 230 grams of NH_3
b. 280 grams of NH_3
c. 2300 grams of NH_3
d. 2800 grams of NH_3

Explanation
Choice *D* is the correct answer.

The following roadmap can be used to determine the produced amount of ammonia gas:

$$Mass \: of \: H_2 \rightarrow Moles \: of \: H_2 \rightarrow Moles \: of \: NH_3 \rightarrow Mass \: of \: NH_3$$

Setting up the equation:

$$500. \: g \: H_2 \times \left(\frac{1 \: Mole \: H_2}{2.02 \: g \: H_2}\right) \times \left(\frac{2 \: Moles \: NH_3}{3 \: Moles \: H_2}\right) \times \left(\frac{17.0 \: g \: NH_3}{1 \: Mole \: NH_3}\right) = 28\underline{0}5.28$$

$$= 2800 \: g \: NH_3$$

115

The molar masses are first obtained by using the periodic table. For example, the molar mass of H_2 is 2.02 grams (2×1.008); by summing the masses of each element in the compound, the molar mass of ammonia is found to be 17.0 g/mol). And finally, the answer is specific to three significant figures, which come from the initial amount of H_2 gas (500 g). Significant figures are not obtained from the unit type expressions. The final answer is rounded down to give 2800 grams of NH_3.

Oxidation and Reduction

In oxidation-reduction (redox) reactions, electrons move from one reactant to the other. One example is the reaction of aluminum (Al) foil in a copper (II) chloride ($CuCl_2$) solution, which produces copper (Cu) and aluminum chloride ($AlCl_3$).

$$2\,Al(s) + 3\,CuCl_2(aq) \xrightarrow{acid} 2\,AlCl_3(aq) + 3Cu(s)$$

Copper (II) chloride ($CuCl_2$) solution has a bluish color that gradually disappears to colorless clear when reacting with aluminum. In the reaction equation, Al is oxidized and loses three electrons (3 e⁻). In inorganic chemistry, **oxidation** is the half-reaction resulting in the loss of electrons by an atom, and **reduction** is the other half-reaction that results in an atom gaining electrons. The lost electrons are then transferred to Cu, which is reduced to form a solid. **Oxidation numbers** are hypothetical charges assigned to an atom based on the actual charge of the atom. These numbers are helpful for keeping track of electrons and are written with a sign followed by a number (e.g., -2, +2). Ions in solution have charges and are written as superscripts with the number followed by a sign

116

(e.g., Al^{3+}). The table below lists the rules for assigning oxidation numbers to elements and ions.

Type	Oxidation number (ox #)	Exceptions
Elements	0	None
Monatomic ions	Group 1A: +1 for Li^+, Na^+ Group 2A: +2 for Mg^{2+}, +3 for Al^{3+}	None
Hydrogen	+1 in most compounds (nonmetals)	-1 in hydrides (compounds with metals, CaH_2)
Halogens (e.g., F^-)	-1 for F^-, Br^-, I^-	Different values when bonded to oxygen or another halogen
Oxygen	-2 in most compounds	-1 in H_2O_2, takes other values when bonded to F
Compounds / ions	The sum of oxidation # is zero (e.g., Fe_2O_3)	Ox # equal to the charge on polyatomic anion: $C_2H_3O_2^- = -1$, $SO_4^{2-} = -2$, $CO_3^{2-} = -2$, $PO_4^{3-} = -3$, $OH^- = -1$

For example, oxidation numbers can be assigned to the reaction of Al and Cu as follows:

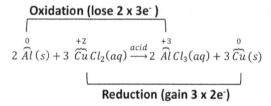

Al(s) is a pure element and will have an oxidation number of zero. Cl will have an oxidation number of -1. Because there are two Cl atoms, the oxidation number of Cu must be +2, because the sum of the oxidation numbers must be zero: $2 \times -1\ (Cl) + 1 \times +2\ (Cu) = 0$. For the AlCl$_3$ compound, the oxidation number for Al is +3, and it is -1 for Cl. The pure Cu element will have an oxidation number of zero. Cu acts as the **oxidizing agent** because it oxidizes another substance (Al), and Al acts as a **reducing agent** because it reduces another substance (Cu). The number of electrons lost on the reactants' side must be equal to the number electrons gained by the products' side. Al is oxidized and loses three electrons. Cu is reduced and gains two electrons. Because there are two Al, this accounts for six lost electrons, which are gained by three Cu atoms.

In the following reaction, which element is oxidized and which is reduced?

$$Fe(s) + CuSO_4(aq) \rightarrow FeSO_4(aq) + Cu(s)$$

a. Fe is reduced and loses electrons, Cu is oxidized and gains electrons.

b. Fe is reduced and gains electrons, Cu is oxidized and loses electrons.

c. Fe is oxidized and loses electrons, Cu is reduced and gains electrons.

d. Fe is oxidized and gains electrons, Cu is reduced and loses electrons.

Explanation

Choice *C* is the correct answer. Oxidation is always the loss of electrons, while reduction is the gain of one or more electrons. This fact, which must be memorized, eliminates Choices *B* and *D*. In this equation, Fe is oxidized (loses 2 electrons) to Fe^{2+} and acts as a reducing agent to Cu^{2+}. Cu^{2+} is reduced (gains two electrons) to form Cu.

Acids and Bases

Acid-base reactions involve proton transfer from an acid to a base. Examples of acids include citric acid ($H_3C_6H_5O_7$) found in lemon juice, and phosphoric acid (H_3PO_4), found in some canned sodas, both which prevent bacteria growth. An **Arrhenius acid** is a molecule that dissolves in water, which results in the creation of protons (H^+). Some acids are strong acids that ionize entirely in water as indicated by the forward reaction arrow ($\rightarrow$). Strong acids are strong electrolytes. The reaction of hydroiodic acid in water produces H^+ and I^-.

$$HI\ (aq) \xrightarrow{H_2O} H^+(aq) + I^-(aq)$$

Drain and household cleaners include bases such as sodium hydroxide (NaOH) and ammonia (NH_3). A molecule that dissolves in water to create a hydroxide ion (OH^-) is an Arrhenius base. Strong bases are strong electrolytes that ionize entirely in water. For example, calcium hydroxide ($Ca(OH)_2$) dissolves in water completely to produce hydroxide ions:

$$Ca(OH)_2\ (aq) \xrightarrow{H_2O} 2OH^-(aq) + Ca^{2+}(aq)$$

The table below lists common strong acids and bases.

Strong Acids		Strong Bases	
$HClO_4$	Perchloric acid	LiOH	Lithium hydroxide
HBr	Hydrobromic acid	$Ca(OH)_2$	Calcium hydroxide
H_2SO_4	Sulfuric acid	NaOH	Sodium hydroxide
HI	Hydroiodic acid	KOH	Potassium hydroxide
HCl	Hydrochloric acid	$Sr(OH)_2$	Strontium hydroxide
HNO_3	Nitric acid	$Ba(OH)_2$	Barium hydroxide

Acids and bases that are not listed in the table above are classified as weak electrolytes. A weak acid, such as acetic acid ($HC_2H_3O_2$), partially ionizes in water as indicated by forward and reverse arrows $\rightleftarrows$. Water acts as the base and accepts a proton from the acetic acid molecule ($HC_2H_3O_2$). The forward

arrow is shorter than the reverse arrow and indicates partial
ionization.

H⁺

$HC_2H_3O_2$ *(aq)* + H_2O *(l)* $\rightleftharpoons$ $C_2H_3O_2^-$ *(aq)* + H_3O^+ *(aq)*
  acid   base

Ammonia (NH_3) is an example of a weak base that partially
ionizes in water. **Neutralization reactions** are another type of
acid-base reaction that yields an ionic compound (salt) and
water. Consider the reaction of hydrochloric acid (HCl) and
potassium hydroxide (KOH), which produces potassium
chloride (salt, KCl) and water (H_2O). The reaction is an exchange
or double replacement reaction whereby the cation of one
species combines with the anion of another species (e.g., H^+ + $^-$
OH)

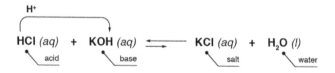

H⁺

HCl *(aq)* + KOH *(aq)* $\rightleftharpoons$ KCl *(aq)* + H_2O *(l)*
  acid   base   salt   water

Question
Imagine that nitric acid is added to water. Which of the
following would be true?

    a. Forward and reverse arrows $\rightleftharpoons$ would be used when
    writing the equation.

    b. The concentration of OH⁻ in the water would increase.

    c. The nitric acid would act as an Arrhenius base.

    d. The nitric acid would completely ionize in the water.

The correct answer is Choice *D*. Nitric acid (HNO_3) is a strong acid, as it is listed in the table. As such, it will completely ionize in water and increase the concentration of H^+ in the water (not OH^-, so Choice *B* is incorrect). Like Choice *B*, Choice *C* also describes a base, not an acid, so it is incorrect. Choice *A* is incorrect because it describes a weak acid (or base), and its partial ionization in water, but nitric acid is a strong one.

Nuclear Chemistry

The energy associated with nuclear reactions is considered millions of times greater compared to that of chemical reactions. Nuclear processes are desirable for space exploration. In 2018, NASA recently demonstrated a new nuclear fission system, which can power human outposts or space exploration on the moon and Mars. Rutherford's atomic theory showed that the atom contains a dense positive nucleus surrounded by electrons. The nucleus or nuclide consists of neutrons and protons. Many nuclei are radioactive and decompose to produce one or more particles. These decay processes fall into two categories: nuclides that show a mass change and nuclide decay processes that do not change mass.

The radioactive decay of Uranium-238 is an example of the first case where the mass of the nuclei changes and produces heavy nuclides such as thorium-234:

$$_{192}^{238}U \rightarrow {}_2^4He + {}_{90}^{234}Th$$

The reaction produces a light **alpha (α) particle** or a helium nucleus (${}_2^4He$) and is a common type of decay for heavy radioactive nuclides. The atomic number (Z) and (A) are conserved. For instance, on the product side, the sum of A for each component is A = 4 + 234 = 238, which is equal to A for uranium-238, A = 238. The sum of Z on the product side is Z = 2 + 90 = 92, which is equivalent to Z for uranium-238, Z = 192.

The second scenario is a common decay process in which the mass remains constant. The decomposition of carbon-14 yields an electron ($_{-1}^{0}e$) called a **beta (β) particle.**

$$^{14}_{6}C \rightarrow {}^{14}_{7}N + {}^{0}_{-1}e$$

The mass number (A) and atomic number (Z) are conserved on both sides of the equation. On the product side Z = 7 + -1 = 6, which is equal to Z for the carbon atom, Z = 6. The mass number for product side A = 14 + 0 = 14, which is equal to the mass number for carbon-14, A = 14. The beta (β) particle has a mass of zero because its mass is relatively small compared to a proton or neutron. Note that Z = -1 for the β particle, which results in a new nuclide having an additional proton, Z = 6 + 1 = 7 ($^{14}_{7}N$). Therefore, β particle production changes a proton to a neutron.

Question
Which of the following regarding alpha particles is true?
  a. Their mass is greater than that of protons and neutrons
  b. Their mass is less than that of beta particles
  c. They have the greatest tissue penetration power
  d. They are high-energy electrons

Explanation
Choice A is correct. The mass of alpha particles is several times greater than the mass of a proton or neutron. It is several thousand times greater than the mass of a beta particle, so

Choice *B* is wrong. Because they are so large, their tissue penetration power is quite low. In fact, just a thick sheet of paper or clothes are enough to stop them and protect the body from penetration; thus, Choice *C* is incorrect. It is beta particles, not alpha, that are high-energy electrons.

Biochemistry

Biochemistry is the study of chemistry in living systems and is vital to understanding how cells create the molecules that are fundamental to life. At least thirty elements are essential to life. The human body is composed of oxygen (sixty-five percent by mass) followed by carbon (eighteen percent by mass). Oxygen is the main component of water and carbon is a component of all organic compounds. Hydrogen and nitrogen make up approximately ten and three percent of the body by mass, and the remaining percentage (mostly less than one percent) is composed of a handful of trace elements.

The molecules of biological organisms fall into four categories: carbohydrates, lipids, nucleic acids, and proteins. **Carbohydrates** serve as an energy source and structural material in plants. For example, fructose is an important carbohydrate or sugar found in fruit and honey. Cells contain water-insoluble substances called **lipids.** One class of lipids is called **fats**, which are esters of glycerol called triglycerides (as shown in the figure below). The three R groups may be the same or different saturated or unsaturated hydrocarbons ($CH3(CH_2)x$-, X is a positive integer). Soap is created by the reaction of sodium hydroxide (NaOH) and triglycerides, a process called **saponification,** which produces glycerol and a fatty acid salt. **Nucleic acids** are responsible for storing and transmitting genetic information. Deoxyribonucleic acid (DNA) is composed of two polymer strands, or high molecular weight substances, made up of repeating units or monomers, which contain a phosphate group, a five-carbon sugar (deoxyribose), and a nitrogen-containing base such as thymine. These three units form a nucleotide or monomer. **Proteins** are made up of different combinations of twenty amino acids that have a central carbon atom bonded to either polar or nonpolar side chains. There are many types of proteins, and each has many functions. For example, muscle and nails are examples of fibrous proteins that provide structural support in humans and animals. Protein chains may either be hydrophilic (water-loving, polar) or hydrophobic (water-fearing, nonpolar). Proteins are assembled when two or more amino acids combine through a condensation reaction. The reaction creates a C-N covalent linkage between a carboxyl group (-COOH) and an amine group (NH_2) of two different molecules. A water molecule is created by the reaction of the -CO<u>OH</u> and N<u>H</u>$_2$ groups.

Carbohydrates

Fructose

CH_2OH
|
$C = O$
|
$HO - C - H$
|
$H - C - OH$
|
$H - C - OH$
|
CH_2OH

Lipids

Triglycerides

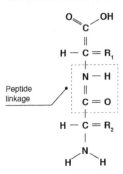

$$H_2C - O - \overset{\overset{\displaystyle O}{\|}}{C} = R_1$$

$$HC - O - \overset{\overset{\displaystyle O}{\|}}{C} - R_2$$

$$H_2C - O - \overset{\overset{\displaystyle O}{\|}}{C} - R_3$$

Nucleic acids

Ribose

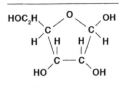

Thymine (T) DNA

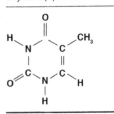

Phosphoric acid

H_3PO_4

Proteins

$$O = \overset{\displaystyle C - OH}{}$$
$$\|$$
$$H - C = R_1$$
|
N — H
‖
C = O
|
$H - C = R_2$
|
N
H   H

Peptide linkage

126

Question

Which of the following statements regarding proteins is FALSE?

a. Two amino acids combine through a condensation reaction.

b. The twenty amino acids differ by their side chains, but all include a central carbon atom.

c. Two amino acids bond together at their amine groups.

d. Protein chains may either be hydrophilic or hydrophobic.

Explanation

The correct answer choice is *C*. While the other three statements about proteins are true, it is not true that two amino acids bond together at their amine groups. Proteins are assembled when two or more amino acids combine through a condensation reaction. The reaction creates a C-N covalent linkage (peptide bonds) between a carboxyl group (-COOH) and an amine group (NH_2) of two different molecules rather than the amine group of both amino acids.

Anatomy and Physiology

General Terminology

Becoming familiar with the terms associated with anatomy and physiology can aid in the understanding of these fields. Anatomy is the study of body parts, both internal and external, and how they relate to each other. Physiology is the study of the function of these body parts, as well as the function of living organisms as a whole. The terminology of anatomy and physiology makes clear which area of the body is being studied.

The table below describes the three main body positions.

Body Position	Description
Anatomical	Person is standing with legs together, feet flat on the floor, and hands at the sides with palms facing forward
Supine	Person is lying down, face up, hands at the sides with palms facing downward
Prone	Person is lying face down, hands at the sides with palms facing upward

The figure below shows the directional terms used to describe the relationship between areas of the body.

Directional terms

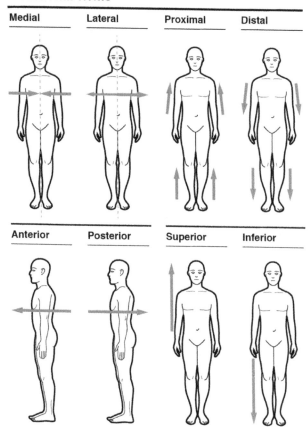

Medial	Lateral	Proximal	Distal

Anterior	Posterior	Superior	Inferior

129

The figure below shows some terms used to refer to different areas of the body. The anatomical term is in parentheses after the name of the body part.

Anterior view

Head   *cephalic*

Forehead	*frontal*	**Nose**	*nasal*
Eye	*orbital*	**Mouth**	*oral*
Cheek	*buccal*	**Chin**	*mental*
Ear	*otic*		

Neck   *cervical*

Trunk

Upper limb

Armpit	*axillary*	**Chest**	*thoracic*
Arm	*brachial*	**Breast**	*mammary*
Front of elbow	*antecubital*	**Abdomen**	*abdominal*
Forearm	*oral*	**Navel**	*ombilical*
Wrist	*carpal*	**Hip**	*coxal*
Hand *manual*			
Palm	*palmar*		
Fingers *digital*			

Lower limb

Thigh	*femoral*	**Pelvis**	*pelvic*
Anterior surface of the knee	*patellar*	**Pubis**	*pubic*
Leg	*crural*	**Groin**	*inguinal*
Foot	*pedal*		
Ankle	*tarsal*		
Toes	*digital*		

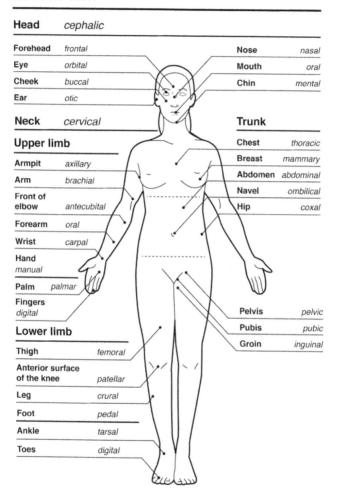

Posterior view

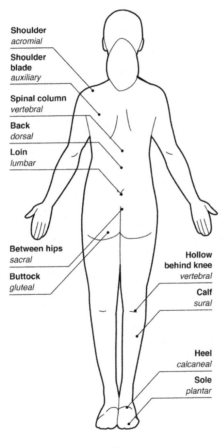

Shoulder
acromial

Shoulder blade
auxiliary

Spinal column
vertebral

Back
dorsal

Loin
lumbar

Between hips
sacral

Buttock
gluteal

Hollow behind knee
vertebral

Calf
sural

Heel
calcaneal

Sole
plantar

Question

If a patient is having lower back pain, which term could they use to describe the area of their pain?

- a. Pedal
- b. Lumbar
- c. Axillary
- d. Cephalic

Explanation

The best answer is Choice *B*. The figure above describes the anatomical terms used for different body parts. In the picture on the right, the lower back is referred to as lumbar, so the patient could refer to their ailment as lumbar pain. Choice *A* would describe foot pain. Choice *C* would describe pain in the arms. Choice *D* would describe pain in a person's head.

Histology

There are 200 different types of cells in the human body. Histology is the study of these different types of cells. Cells group together to form tissues, and tissue group together to form organs. Organs have specialized functions in the body that are vital for living. The four primary types of tissue are epithelial, connective, muscle, and neural. Epithelial tissue lines internal body cavities and passages and covers exposed surfaces. This type of tissue does not contain blood vessels. Connective tissue fills internal spaces and creates a protective barrier for organs. Muscle tissue is contractile and helps with movement of the body. It also helps maintain posture and control body temperature. Neural tissue is concentrated in the brain and spinal cord. It conducts electrical impulses that help send information throughout the body.

Question
Patient A has sores along the inside of her mouth. Which type of tissue is most likely damaged?

    a. Muscle

    b. Neural

    c. Connective

    d. Epithelial

Explanation
The best answer is Choice *D*. Using histology to look for cell damage in the epithelial tissue lining the mouth, such as along the inner walls of the cheeks, could explain why the patient is getting sores and having pain. Muscle, neural, and connective tissues, Choices *A*, *B*, and *C*, have different functions in the body and tend to be located in higher concentration in areas other than the lining of the mouth. Mouth sores would most likely be due to epithelial tissue damage.

Mitosis and Meiosis

Mitosis and meiosis are two different ways in which cells replicate and divide. Most cells in the body undergo mitosis, which helps to replace damaged and dying cells. An individual cell replicates its genetic material and then divides into two identical daughter cells. Meiosis is a more complicated replication process that occurs in gamete cells, or reproductive cells. In meiosis, two non-identical parent gamete cells combine and replicate their genetic material, or chromosomes, and then undergo two phases of division. Human gamete cells each have 23 chromosomes. When a sperm cell combines with an egg cell, the resulting diploid cell has 46 chromosomes. These 46 chromosomes replicate themselves and then also cross over so that the genes are mixed up. After the first division process, there are two daughter cells with 46 chromosomes each. After the second division process, there are four daughter cells with 23 chromosomes each. However, unlike in mitosis, the daughter cells are NOT identical to either of their parent cells because of the crossing over that occurs before cell division starts.

The figure below depicts the steps of cell replication and division by mitosis.

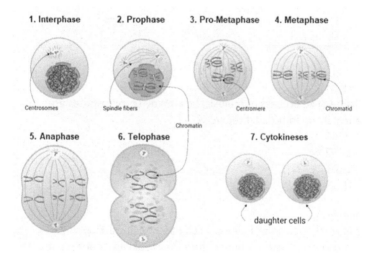

The figure below depicts cell replication and division by meiosis.

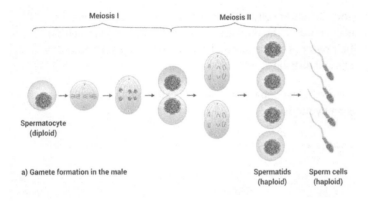

a) Gamete formation in the male

Question
Following the process of meiosis, how many chromosomes are in each of the four daughter cells?

    a. 46

    b. 92

    c. 23

    d. 13

Explanation
The correct answer is Choice *C*. Each parent cell starts with 23 chromosomes. They combine before they replicate to form one cell that has 46 chromosomes, Choice *A*. After they replicate, there are 92 chromosomes, Choice *B*, in the cell. After both division processes, when meiosis is complete, the daughter cells end up with the same number of chromosomes as each individual parent, which is 23 chromosomes.

Skin

The skin provides a barrier for the body from variations in temperature and mechanical impacts. It also helps protect the body from microorganisms and chemicals. The skin contains sweat glands that help to regulate internal temperature and remove waste by pulling water and sodium salts to the surface of the body. It also contains sebaceous glands that secrete **sebum**, an oily mixture of lipids and proteins that protects the skin from bacterial and fungal infections.

The Sun can have a detrimental effect on unprotected skin. After a short period of exposure time, ultraviolet (UV) rays can cause damage to the DNA of skin cells. Cells are equipped to repair the damage before continuing their replication and division process, but if the damage is too severe, the cells undergo apoptosis so that the DNA damage is not passed on to daughter cells. If the damage is passed on, diseases such as skin cancer may develop.

Question
Which option would NOT help a person protect their skin cells from damage?

    a. Sitting in the shade instead of directly under the sun
    b. Sitting directly under the Sun
    c. Applying sunscreen as a barrier to UV ray absorption
    d. Wearing a hat to provide shade to their head and face

Explanation
The best answer is Choice *B*. Skin cells are susceptible to damage when exposed directly to the sun. Choices *A*, *C*, and *D* all provide protection to the skin cells from direct exposure to

the Sun. In the shade, there is no direct exposure to the UV rays from the sun. Sunscreen provides a layer of protection between the sun and skin cells.

Skeletal System

The skeletal system comprises the 206 bones of the skeleton and the ligaments, cartilage, and connective tissue that connect and stabilize them. This system forms protective barriers around delicate organs. For example, the ribs protect the heart and lungs, and the vertebrae protect the spinal cord. The skeleton also provides a framework for muscles and other soft tissue to attach to. Bones are strong and hard to break because of the calcium salts and collagen fibers that make them up. The calcium salts provide strength while the collagen fibers provide flexibility. Two types of bone make up the skeleton: compact and spongy. Compact bone is dense and filled with organic ground substance and inorganic salts. Spongy bone is porous and lightweight. The spongy bone covers the compact bone in an open framework.

The figure on the next page shows the names of different bones in the skeleton.

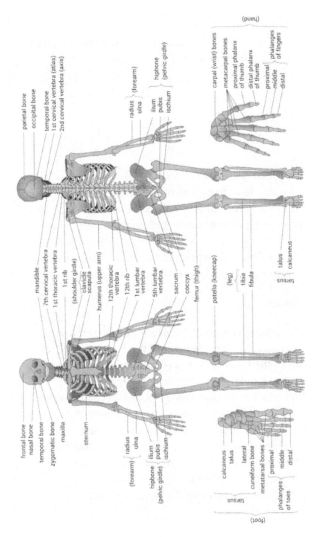

parietal bone
occipital bone
temporal bone
1st cervical vertebra (atlas)
2nd cervical vertebra (axis)

radius } (forearm)
ulna

ilium
pubis } hipbone (pelvic girdle)
ischium

(hand)

carpal (wrist) bones
metacarpal bones
proximal phalanx of thumb
distal phalanx of thumb
proximal
middle } phalanges of fingers
distal

mandible
7th cervical vertebra
1st thoracic vertebra
1st rib
clavicle } (shoulder girdle)
scapula
humerus (upper arm)
12th thoracic vertebra
12th rib
1st lumbar vertebra
5th lumbar vertebra
sacrum
coccyx
femur (thigh)
patella (kneecap)
tibia } (leg)
fibula
talus
calcaneus } tarsus

frontal bone
nasal bone
temporal bone
zygomatic bone
maxilla
sternum
radius } (forearm)
ulna
ilium
pubis } hipbone (pelvic girdle)
ischium

calcaneus
talus
lateral cuneiform bone
metatarsal bones
proximal
middle } phalanges of toes
distal
tarsus
(foot)

139

If a person falls and hits their head, which part of the skeleton protects their brain from injury?

a. Pelvic girdle
b. Ribs
c. Vertebrae
d. Cranium

Explanation

The correct answer is Choice *D*. The skeletal system provides protection for the delicate organs of the body. The brain is located in the head; the cranium—also called the skull—is the bony structure that provides protection to the head. The pelvic girdle, Choice *A*, supports the hips and protects the inner organs. The ribs, Choice *B*, protect the lungs and heart in the chest. The vertebrae, Choice *C*, protect the spinal cord.

Muscular System

The muscular system comprises approximately 700 muscles, which are responsible for movement of the body. The muscles are attached to the bones of the skeletal system by tendons, which are dense bands of connective tissue made up of collagen fibers. There are three types of muscle tissue: skeletal, cardiac, and smooth. Skeletal tissue aids in movement of the body by pulling on the bones of the skeleton. Cardiac tissue makes up the heart and helps to pump blood back and forth in the body through the arteries and veins. Smooth muscle tissue helps with movement in many other body systems, including moving food and liquids through the digestive tract.

All muscle tissue has the following four properties:

- It is excitable, which means it responds to stimuli.

- It is contractile, which means the muscle shortens and pulls on the attached connective tissue.

- It is extensible, which means it can be stretched.

- It is elastic, which means it can return to its original length after being extended.

Question

Which characteristic of muscle tissue describes its ability to shorten?

a. Contractility
b. Excitability
c. Elasticity
d. Extensibility

Explanation

The correct answer is Choice *A*. Contractility describes the ability of muscles to shorten, which can cause movement of the skeleton. Choice *B*, excitability, describes the ability of muscles to respond to stimuli. Choice *C*, elasticity, describes how muscles return to their original length after being stretched. Choice *D*, extensibility, describes the ability of muscles to lengthen.

Nervous System

The nervous system controls and adjusts the activities of all of the other systems in the body. It is divided into two systems:

the central nervous system (CNS), which consists of the brain and spinal cord, and the peripheral nervous system (PNS), which consists of the remaining neural tissue. The CNS is in charge of processing and coordinating motor commands and sensory data. It also processes intelligence, learning, emotions, and memory. The PNS transmits sensory information between the CNS and other systems in the body. The PNS is also further subdivided into afferent and efferent divisions. The afferent division transmits sensory information from the body back to the CNS. The efferent division transmits motor commands to the muscles and glands of the body. It comprises the somatic nervous system, which is in charge of skeletal muscle contractions, and the autonomic nervous system, which controls smooth muscle, cardiac muscle, and gland activity.

Question

Which part of the nervous system controls activity of the heart?

    a. CNS

    b. Afferent division

    c. Autonomic nervous system

    d. Somatic nervous system

Explanation

The correct answer is Choice *C*. The heart itself is made up of cardiac muscle tissue, and the autonomic nervous system controls activity of cardiac muscle. The CNS, Choice *A*, comprises the brain and spinal cord. The afferent division of the PNS, Choice *B*, is responsible for transmitting sensory information to the CNS. The somatic nervous system, Choice *D*, controls skeletal muscle contractions.

Endocrine System

The endocrine system works closely with the nervous system to maintain homeostasis in the body by regulating the activities of the other systems. The ductless tissues and glands that make up the endocrine system secrete hormones into the interstitial fluids of the body. Hormones are chemicals that affect the metabolism of specific organs and tissues.

The table below lists the major glands that are part of the endocrine system and their functions:

Gland	Function
Pituitary gland	Releases hormones that regulate growth, blood pressure, internal temperature, and pain
Hypothalamus	Connects the endocrine system to the nervous system through the pituitary gland
Thyroid gland	Releases hormones that are critical for brain development during infancy and childhood, metabolism, growth and development, temperature regulation, and regulation of the amount of circulating calcium
Parathyroid gland	Releases parathyroid hormone, which aids the thyroid in regulating the amount of calcium in circulation
Adrenal glands	Aids in the management of stress
Thymus gland	Releases hormones that are important for development and maintenance of regular immunological defenses

Pineal gland	Releases melatonin, which can slow the maturation of the reproductive organs and gamete cells; regulates the body's circadian rhythm, which is the wake-sleep cycle
Pancreas	Regulates blood sugar in the body

Question

Which endocrine gland helps regulate the amount of sleep a person gets?

    a. Pancreas

    b. Pineal gland

    c. Parathyroid gland

    d. Hypothalamus

Explanation

The best answer is Choice *B*. The pineal gland regulates the circadian rhythm, which is the body's wake-sleep cycle. The pancreas, Choice *A*, regulates blood sugar. The parathyroid gland, Choice *C*, helps regulate the amount of calcium in the blood. The hypothalamus, Choice *D*, connects the endocrine system to the nervous system.

Circulatory System

The circulatory system comprises the heart and blood vessels of the body. The heart pumps blood to the rest of the body through the blood vessels. The circulating blood brings oxygen, nutrients, and hormones to all the cells in the body through arteries. Veins bring oxygen-depleted blood back to the heart. This exchange keeps all of the tissues and organs thriving and healthy. Blood is made up of red blood cells, which transport oxygen and carbon dioxide; white blood cells, which help fight off diseases; and platelets, which contain factors that help with blood clotting.

Heart rate can be measured using a stethoscope. A stethoscope has a round plastic diaphragm that is placed on the chest, over the heart. When the heart beats, a sound occurs and makes a vibration. When someone is using a stethoscope, the vibration of the heartbeat travels through a hollow tube in the stethoscope to the earpiece. A sphygmomanometer is used to measure blood pressure. An inflatable cuff is placed around the arm and is used to collapse and release an artery in a controlled manner to determine the pressure of the blood flowing through the artery.

Question
Which instrument is used to measure a person's heart rate?
- a. Sphygmomanometer
- b. Otoscope
- c. Syringe
- d. Stethoscope

Explanation
The correct answer is Choice *D*. A stethoscope transmits the vibrations from the heartbeat to an earpiece so that the rate of beating can be measured. A sphygmomanometer, Choice *A*, measures blood pressure. An otoscope, Choice *B*, is used to look in a person's ears. A syringe, Choice *C*, can be used to deliver medicine to the body.

Respiratory System

The respiratory system is responsible for the act of breathing, which enables the exchange of gases between the air and blood. This system can be divided into the upper and lower respiratory systems. The upper system comprises the nose, nasal cavity, sinuses, and pharynx. The lower system comprises the larynx, trachea, small passageways leading to the lungs (called the bronchi and then smaller bronchioles), and the lungs. When air is inhaled, oxygen from the air enters the nose or mouth, passes into the sinuses where temperature and humidity are regulated, and then enters the trachea where it is filtered. Next, the air travels through the bronchi, which are lined with cilia and mucus to further filter the air of germs and dust. Finally, the air reaches the lungs. There, in the small sacs called alveoli, oxygen from the inspired air is exchanged with carbon dioxide in the blood in the pulmonary capillaries. Carbon dioxide is exhaled through the nose or mouth while the now oxygen-rich blood is transported to the heart, ready to be circulated to the rest of the body.

Question

Which of the following is a part of the lower respiratory system?

   a. Sinuses
   b. Trachea
   c. Nose
   d. Pharynx

Explanation

The correct answer is Choice *B*. The trachea is a part of the lower respiratory system, along with the larynx, the small passageways leading to the lungs (the bronchi and bronchioles), and the lungs. The trachea helps to filter inhaled air that is traveling to the lungs. The sinuses, nose, and pharynx, Choices *A*, *C*, and *D*, are all part of the upper respiratory system.

Digestive System

The digestive system converts food and fluids to energy that the body can use as fuel for activities. It comprises a group of organs that work together to complete this transformation. Food and fluids are ingested through the mouth and then pass through the gastrointestinal (GI) tract. Different organs help with the breakdown of the foods and the absorption of nutrients. Waste products are then eliminated from the body.

The table below summarizes the different steps involved in the digestive process:

Step	Description
Ingestion	Food and fluids enter the mouth and the alimentary canal
Mechanical processing	The teeth tear up the food and the tongue aids in swallowing the processed food
Digestion	Chemicals and enzymes break down the food into smaller molecules that can be absorbed by the digestive epithelium
Secretion	Organs secrete acids, buffers, and enzymes to further aid in breakdown of the food
Absorption	The digestive epithelium absorbs vitamins, electrolytes, water, and organic molecules from the food and fluids
Compaction	Materials that are indigestible and waste products are dehydrated and compacted together into feces
Excretion	Waste products are secreted into the digestive tract for removal from the body

The figure below depicts the organs of the digestive system.

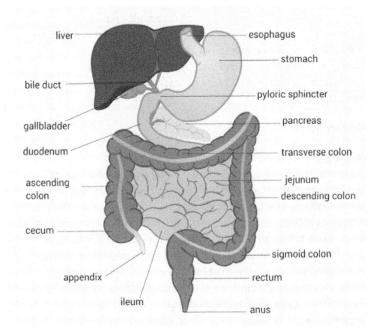

Question
During which step of digestion do the teeth tear up food that has entered the mouth?

    a. Secretion

    b. Absorption

    c. Excretion

    d. Mechanical processing

The correct answer is Choice *D*. In mechanical processing the teeth tear up large chunks of food into smaller pieces. In secretion, Choice *A*, buffers, enzymes, and acids are secreted to help break complex molecules into simpler ones. In absorption, Choice *B*, nutrients are absorbed through the digestive epithelium. In excretion, Choice *C*, waste products are removed from the body.

Urinary System

Summary
The urinary system is responsible for excreting organic waste products, excess water, and electrolytes that are generated by other systems. The organs that comprise this system are the kidneys, ureters, urinary bladder, and urethra. The kidneys filter waste products out of the blood. They contain millions of tiny filtering units called nephrons. The nephrons take out fluid and waste products from the blood to produce urine. Large molecules and blood cells are too big to pass through the nephrons; they remain in the blood. Once urine has accumulated, it is passed into the ureters and then into the urinary bladder. The urinary bladder is hollow and very elastic. As the volume of urine increases in the urinary bladder, the walls stretch and become thinner to relieve any build-up of internal pressure. When the body is ready for urination, the muscles of the urinary bladder contract and push the urine through the urethra and out of the body.

Question
Which organ is responsible for filtering waste products out of the blood?

    a. Ureter
    b. Kidney
    c. Urethra
    d. Urinary bladder

Explanation
The correct answer is Choice *B*. The kidneys contain millions of nephrons that filter waste products and fluids out of the blood to produce urine. Larger molecules and blood cells remain in the blood. The urinary bladder, Choice *D*, is where urine is stored as it accumulates in the body. The ureters and the urethra, Choices *A* and *C*, are passages that transport the urine to the urinary bladder and out of the body, respectively.

Reproductive System

The reproductive system is made up of the reproductive organs (called gonads), reproductive tract, accessory glands, and external genitalia. This system produces, stores, nourishes, and transports functional reproductive cells. The male and female reproductive systems are different from each other. The male gonads are the testes, which secrete testosterone and produce sperm cells, the male reproductive cells. The female gonads are the ovaries, which secrete estrogen and progesterone and produce oocytes, the female reproductive cells. During the process of human reproduction, sperm cells are expelled from the male reproductive system into the female reproductive system, where they then fertilize an oocyte in the uterus. The resulting embryo embeds itself into the uterine wall and develops for nine months before it is ready for the outside world.

The figure below shows the male and female reproductive systems.

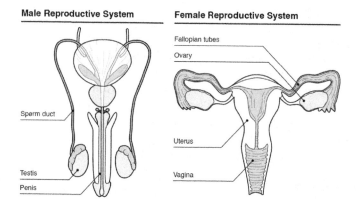

Male Reproductive System

Sperm duct

Testis

Penis

Female Reproductive System

Fallopian tubes

Ovary

Uterus

Vagina

Question

Oocytes are produced by the ovaries. Which part of the reproductive system must an oocyte travel through before being fertilized by a sperm cell?

    a. Penis

    b. Sperm duct

    c. Fallopian tube

    d. Vagina

Explanation

The correct answer is Choice *C*. As shown in the figure, the fallopian tubes are the passageway between the ovaries and the uterus. The penis, Choice *A*, is the part of the male reproductive system from which the sperm cells are expelled. The sperm cells travel through the sperm duct, Choice *B*. The vagina, Choice *D*, is part of the female reproductive system but is not between the ovaries and the uterus.

Dear HESI Test Taker,

We would like to start by thanking you for purchasing this study guide for your HESI exam. We hope that we exceeded your expectations. If you found something not up to your standards, please send us an email and let us know.

We would also like to let you know about other books in our catalog that may interest you.

ATI TEAS 6: amazon.com/dp/162845427X

CEN: amazon.com/dp/1628454768

We have study guides in a wide variety of fields. If the one you are looking for isn't listed above, then try searching for it on Amazon or send us an email.

Thanks Again and Happy Testing!
Product Development Team
info@studyguideteam.com

Interested in buying more than 10 copies of our product? Contact us about bulk discounts:
bulkorders@studyguideteam.com

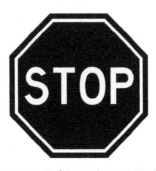

FREE Test Taking Tips DVD Offer

Don't forget that doing well on your exam includes both understanding the test content and understanding how to use what you know to do well on the test. We offer a completely FREE Test Taking Tips DVD that covers world class test taking tips that you can use to be even more successful when you are taking your test.

All that we ask is that you email us your feedback about your study guide. To get your **FREE Test Taking Tips DVD**, email freedvd@studyguideteam.com with "FREE DVD" in the subject line and the following information in the body of the email:

- The title of your study guide.
- Your product rating on a scale of 1-5, with 5 being the highest rating.
- Your feedback about the study guide. What did you think of it?
- Your full name and shipping address to send your free DVD.

Made in the
USA
Monee, IL